Lacerations and
Acute Wounds

An Evidence-Based Guide

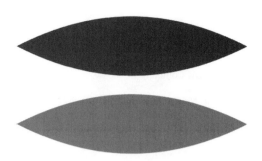

Lacerations and
Acute Wounds
An Evidence-Based Guide

ADAM J. SINGER, MD
Associate Professor of Emergency Medicine
Clinical Research Director
Department of Emergency Medicine
Stony Brook University
Stony Brook, New York

JUDD E. HOLLANDER, MD
Professor
Clinical Research Director
Department of Emergency Medicine
Hospital of University of Pennsylvania
Philadelphia, Pennsylvania

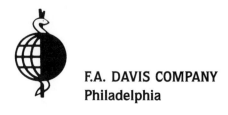

F.A. DAVIS COMPANY
Philadelphia

F. A. Davis Company
1915 Arch Street
Philadelphia, PA 19103
www.fadavis.com

Printed in the United States of America

Last digit indicates print number: 10 9 8 7 6 5 4 3 2 1

Acquisitions Editor: Margaret Biblis
Developmental Editor: Bernice Wissler
Production Editor: Nwakaego Fletcher-Perry
Cover Designer: Louis Forgione

As new scientific information becomes available through basic and clinical research, recommended treatments and drug therapies undergo changes. The author(s) and publisher have done everything possible to make this book accurate, up to date, and in accord with accepted standards at the time of publication. The author(s), editors, and publisher are not responsible for errors or omissions or for consequences from application of the book, and make no warranty, expressed or implied, in regard to the contents of the book. Any practice described in this book should be applied by the reader in accordance with professional standards of care used in regard to the unique circumstances that may apply in each situation. The reader is advised always to check product information (package inserts) for changes and new information regarding dose and contraindications before administering any drug. Caution is especially urged when using new or infrequently ordered drugs.

Library of Congress Cataloging-in-Publication Data

Lacerations and acute wounds / [edited by] Adam J. Singer, Judd E. Hollander.
   p. cm.
  Includes bibliographical references and index.
  ISBN 0-8036-0775-X
   1. Skin—Wounds and injuries.   2. Soft tissue injuries.   3. Wounds and injuries.   4. Wound Healing. I. Singer, Adam J. II. Hollander, Judd E., 1960-

RD93 .L32 2003
617.4'7—dc21

2002024393

PREFACE

Man has cared for cutaneous wounds since the beginning of time. Until recently, most wound care practices were empirical—based on anecdotal clinical experience or animal studies. With the recent emphasis on evidence-based medicine and the development of reliable and validated wound outcome measures, we felt the need for an evidence-based guide for the management of lacerations and other acute cutaneous wounds. Currently there are several fine textbooks that address the care of acute wounds, but most of them are impractical, costly, or represent the personal opinions of their authors.

This text was written by experienced and well-recognized physicians and researchers from several medical specialties, including emergency medicine, plastic surgery, general surgery, dermatology, pediatrics, and infectious diseases. The book is intended as a practical guide for medical students, interns, residents, physician extenders, and attending physicians who care for acute lacerations and surgical incisions as well as other cutaneous wounds.

Most chapters follow a similar format that includes the relevant scientific evidence as well as the advantages, disadvantages, indications, and contraindications for the various wound closure methods. It also identifies many potential pitfalls and includes practical tips that will help achieve optimal wound outcome. To enhance comprehension, much of this information is presented in table format. The book also includes many original figures that help illustrate a number of the wound care practices. We hope that you will find this guide useful.

Adam J. Singer, MD
Stony Brook, New York

Judd E. Hollander, MD
Philadelphia, Pennsylvania

CONTRIBUTORS

Joel M. Bartfield, MD
Residency Director, Emergency Medicine
Albany Medical College
Albany, New York

John S. Brebbia, MD
Assistant Professor of Surgery
Department of Surgery
Stony Brook University
Stony Brook, New York

Richard A. F. Clark, MD
Professor and Chairman of Dermatology
Department of Dermatology
Stony Brook University
Stony Brook, New York

Jose J. Cruz, MD
Associate Clinical Professor of Surgery
Department of Surgery
University of Philippines
Manila, Philippines

Daniel J. Dire, MD, FACEP
Section of Emergency Medicine
Oklahoma University Health Sciences Center
Oklahoma City, Oklahoma

Steven M. Green, MD
Professor of Emergency Medicine and Pediatrics
Loma Linda University Medical Center & Children's Hospital
Loma Linda University School of Medicine
Loma Linda, California

Judd E. Hollander, MD
Professor
Clinical Research Director
Department of Emergency Medicine
Hospital of University of Pennsylvania
Philadelphia, Pennsylvania

Hans R. House, MD
Department of Emergency Medicine and
Department of Internal Medicine
UCLA/Olive View–UCLA Medical Center
Los Angeles, California

Baruch Krauss, MD, EdM
Instructor of Pediatrics
Boston Children's Hospital
Harvard Medical School
Boston, Massachusetts

Richard Lammers, MD
Associate Professor of Emergency Medicine
Michigan State University/Kalamazoo Center for Medical Studies
Kalamazoo, Michigan

Gregory J. Moran, MD
Associate Clinical Professor of Medicine
UCLA School of Medicine
Los Angeles, California
Department of Emergency Medicine and Division of Infectious Diseases
Olive View-UCLA Medical Center
Sylmar, California

Charles V. Pollack, Jr, MD
Chairman, Department of Emergency Medicine
Pennsylvania Hospital
Associate Professor of Emergency Medicine
University of Pennsylvania School of Medicine
Philadelphia, Pennsylvania

James V. Quinn, MD
Associate Clinical Professor of Medicine
Division of Emergency Medicine
University of California Medical Center
San Francisco, California

Lior Rosenberg, MD
Professor and Chair
Department of Plastic Surgery
Ben Gurion University
Beer-Sheba, Israel

Adam J. Singer, MD
Clinical Research Director
Associate Professor of Emergency Medicine
Department of Emergency Medicine
Stony Brook University
Stony Brook, New York

Harry S. Soroff, MD
Professor of Surgery
Department of Surgery
Stony Brook University
Stony Brook, New York

CONTENTS

1. The Biology of Wound Healing
Adam J. Singer, MD, and Richard A. F. Clark, MD   1

2. Patient and Wound Assessment: Basic Concepts of the Patient History and Physical Examination
Judd E. Hollander, MD   9

3. Wound Preparation
Adam J. Singer, MD, and Judd E. Hollander, MD   13

4. Wound Anesthesia
Joel M. Bartfield, MD   23

5. Procedural Sedation and Analgesia
Steven M. Green, MD, and Baruch Krauss, MD, EdM   42

6. Wound Closure Options
Judd E. Hollander, MD   56

7. Adhesive Tapes
Adam J. Singer, MD   64

8. Surgical Staples
Adam J. Singer, MD   73

9. Tissue Adhesives
Adam J. Singer, MD, and James V. Quinn, MD   83

10. Selecting Sutures and Needles for Wound Closure
Judd E. Hollander, MD, and Adam J. Singer, MD   98

11. Basic Suturing and Tissue Handling Techniques
Adam J. Singer, MD, and Lior Rosenberg, MD   108

12. Animal Bites
Daniel J. Dire, MD, FACEP   133

13. Foreign Bodies in Wounds
Richard Lammers, MD   147

14. Plantar Puncture Wounds
Richard Lammers, MD   157

15. Cutaneous and Subcutaneous Abscesses
Charles V. Pollack, Jr., MD   161

16. Burns
Harry S. Soroff, MD; *J. J. Cruz*, MD;
and John S. Brebbia, MD   173

17. Postoperative Care of Wounds
Judd E. Hollander, MD   188

18. Antibiotics in Wound Management
Gregory J. Moran, MD, *and Hans R. House*, MD   194

Index   205

ADAM J. SINGER, MD
RICHARD A. F. CLARK, MD

CHAPTER

1

The Biology of Wound Healing

Wound healing is a complex process that results from interactions between cells, cytokines, and extracellular matrix (ECM).[1] Wound healing has traditionally been divided into several stages, including inflammation, tissue formation, and tissue remodeling, but these phases overlap considerably. For more detail, see Singer and Clark's[2] recent review of the process. Table 1–1 summarizes the sources and actions of various wound cytokines.

STAGES OF HEALING

HEMOSTASIS

Immediately after injury, blood vessels are disrupted, resulting in extravasation of various blood constituents. Reflex vasoconstriction helps reduce blood loss, and platelets begin to aggregate at the site of injury, forming a provisional platelet plug. Tissue injury activates the clotting cascade and a blood clot forms, which stops bleeding.[1] In addition to facilitating the formation of a hemostatic plug, platelets are also responsible for the release of a variety of growth factors (e.g., platelet-derived growth factor [PDGF]) that help attract and activate monocytes and fibroblasts.[3]

INFLAMMATION

Tissue injury also activates the complement system. This results in the release of a variety of chemoattractant agents that recruit neutrophils to the site of injury within the first 12 to 24 hours after injury. The neutrophils help clean any bacteria or foreign debris from the wound.[4] Within 24 to 48 hours, monocytes

TABLE 1–1. CYTOKINES AFFECTING WOUND HEALING

Cytokine	Major Source	Target Cells and Major Effects
Epidermal growth factor family		**Epidermal and mesenchymal regeneration**
EGF	Platelets	Promotes pleiotropic cell motility and proliferation
TGF	Macrophages, epidermal cells	Promotes pleiotropic cell motility and proliferation
Heparin-binding epidermal growth factor	Macrophages	Promotes pleiotropic cell motility and proliferation
Fibroblast growth factor family		**Wound vascularization**
Basic fibroblast growth factor	Macrophages, endothelial cells	Angiogenesis and fibroblast mitogen
Acidic fibroblast growth factor	Macrophages, endothelial cells	Angiogenesis and fibroblast mitogen
Keratinocyte growth factor	Fibroblasts	Promotes epidermal cell motility and proliferation
TGF-β family		**Fibrosis and increased tensile strength**
TGF-β1 and -β2	Platelets, macrophages	Epidermal cell motility, chemotaxis of macrophages and fibroblasts, ECM synthesis and remodeling
TGF-β3	Macrophages	Anti-scarring effects
Other cytokines		
PDGF	Platelets, macrophages, epidermal cells	Fibroblast mitogen and chemoattractant, macrophage chemoattractant and activator
VEGF	Epidermal cells, macrophages	Angiogenesis and increased vascular permeability
TNF	Neutrophils	Pleiotropic growth factor expression
Interleukin-1	Neutrophils	Pleiotropic growth factor expression
Insulin-like growth factor 1	Fibroblasts, epidermal cells	Reepithelialization and granulation tissue formation
CSF 1	Multiple cells	Macrophage activation and granulation tissue formation

CSF = colony-stimulating factor; EGF = epidermal growth factor; TGF = transforming growth factor; TNF = tumor necrosis factor; VEGF = vascular endothelial cell growth factor.

Source: Adapted with permission from Singer, AJ, and Clark, RAF: Cutaneous wound healing. N Engl J Med 341:738–746, 1999.

are also attracted to the wound site. After adherence to components of the ECM, these monocytes undergo metamorphosis and become activated, forming tissue macrophages that play a central role in wound healing.[5] In addition to phagocytosis and ingestion of neutrophils or debris, macrophages also secrete a variety of growth factors such as PDGF, transforming growth factor-β (TGF-β), and vascular endothelial growth factor (VEGF). These help shift the healing process from inflammation to formation of granulation tissue.[6]

RE-EPITHELIALIZATION

The process of re-epithelialization, by which epidermal cells resurface the wound, begins within hours after injury. Epidermal cells, mostly from adjacent skin appendages, begin to migrate and dissect through the wound from the wound edges (Fig. 1–1). This is followed by proliferation of epidermal cells at the wound margin. The exact stimuli for epidermal cell migration and proliferation are unclear. Local release of growth factors (e.g., epidermal growth

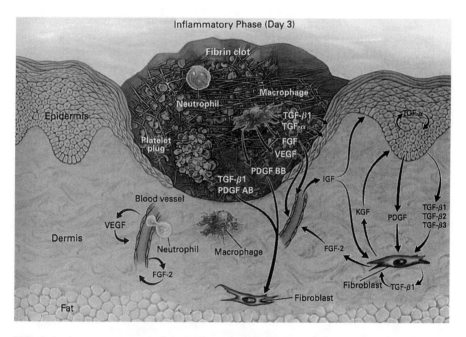

FIG. 1–1. A cutaneous wound three days after injury. Growth factors thought to be necessary for wound healing are shown. KGF = keratinocyte growth factor; TGF-β = transforming growth factor β; IGF = insulin-like growth factor; PDGF = platelet-derived growth factor; TGF-α = transforming growth factor α; VEGF = vascular endothelial cell growth factor; FGF = fibroblast growth factor. (Reprinted with permission from Singer, AJ, and Clark, RAF: Cutaneous wound healing. N Engl J Med 341:738–746, 1999.)

factor, keratinocyte growth factor, and TGF-α) as well as the increased expression of growth factor receptors may help accelerate re-epithelialization.[7,8] Advancement of epidermal cells over the surface of the wound depends on the interaction between specific cell surface receptors (i.e., integrins) and ECM components.[9,10] Degradation of the fibrin clot is also necessary and is facilitated by the release of a variety of matrix metalloproteinases, which are members of a family of zinc-dependent endopeptidases with a broad spectrum of proteolytic activity.[10] With simple lacerations, re-epithelialization may be completed within 1 or 2 days. With more extensive injuries, this process may require several days to weeks. The process of re-epithelialization is enhanced by a moist wound environment.[11]

GRANULATION TISSUE FORMATION

Granulation tissue is composed of blood vessels and fibroblasts, as well as extracellular components. Macrophages, fibroblasts, and blood vessels move into the wounded area as a group.[12] Components of the newly formed ECM provide a scaffold for cell migration as a result of interaction with cell surface receptors.[13] After migrating into the wound, fibroblasts begin synthesizing various elements of the ECM. The fibroblasts also synthesize collagen, perhaps as the result of being stimulated by TGF-β1.[14,15] This collagen gradually replaces the matrix. The fibroblasts eventually stop producing collagen, and a relatively acellular scar replaces the granulation tissue.[16]

NEOVASCULARIZATION

The formation of new blood vessels is a complex process that involves the interaction of cellular components with the ECM and a host of angiogenic factors.[17,18] The process of angiogenesis is necessary to sustain the newly formed granulation tissue. After tissue injury, macrophages and epidermal cells release a variety of cytokines that regulate the formation of new blood vessels. Hypoxia also plays an important role in stimulating neovascularization.[19] Proteolytic enzymes are released that help digest blood vessel basement membranes, allowing migration of endothelial cells to the wound site to form new vessels.[20] After the wound is filled with new vessels, angiogenesis is turned off. This process is probably regulated by a long list of anti-angiogenesis factors such as angiostatin and endostatin.[21]

WOUND CONTRACTION AND REORGANIZATION

As a result of complex interactions between cells, ECM proteins, and cytokines, wound contraction begins approximately 2 weeks after injury. Myofibroblasts, which are modified fibroblasts, are the cells primarily responsible for wound contraction.[22] The process of wound contracture requires attachment of the fibroblasts to the collagen matrix through specialized cell surface receptors (i.e., integrins) under the influence of growth factors such as TGF-β1

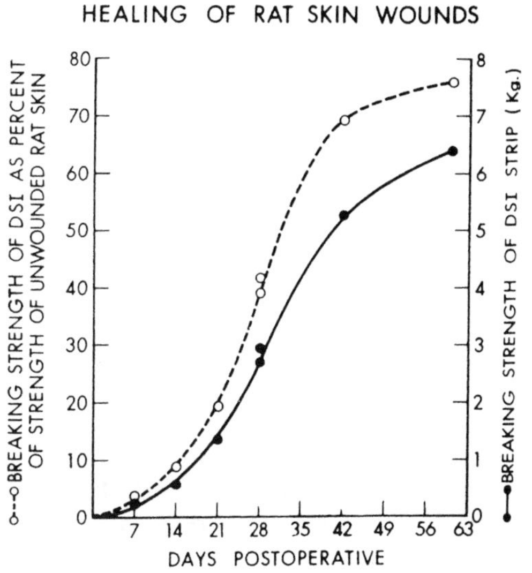

HEALING OF RAT SKIN WOUNDS

FIG. 1–2. Increase in breaking strength of a healing wound shown absolutely and as percent strength of comparable unwounded skin. (Reprinted with permission from Levenson SM, Geever EF, Crowley LV, Oates JF, Berard CW, and Rosen H: The healing of rat skin wounds. Ann Surg 161:293–308, 1965.)

and -β2 and PDGF.[23–25] Maturation of the scar depends on a delicate balance between collagen synthesis and degradation. The degradation is regulated by a set of proteolytic enzymes secreted by macrophages, epidermal cells, and endothelial cells.[26]

During the first 3 weeks of healing, the synthesis of new collagen determines the gain in wound tensile strength. As time goes by, the gain in tensile strength is mostly the result of collagen cross-linking and remodeling. **At 1 week after injury, most wounds have gained only 5 to 10 percent of their original tensile strength. Over the next 6 weeks, most of the original tensile strength is regained, but wounds never attain the same breaking strength as intact skin (Fig. 1–2).**[27] At the end of the first year, most wounded skin is only 70 to 80 percent as strong as unwounded skin.[27]

DETERMINANTS OF COSMETIC OUTCOME

During the first year after injury, the scar continues to mature, so its ultimate appearance may not be evident before this time. Its final appearance depends on both host and environmental factors. The presence of infection at any time may result in poor scarring. Systemic conditions such as diabetes mellitus, deficiency of protein or vitamin C, renal failure, or disorders of collagen or connective tissue formation also may result in suboptimal scars. In addition, the patient's use of systemic corticosteroids, chemotherapeutic agents, or immunosuppressants can also impair healing. The effects of systemic steroids on healing may be partially reversed by administration of vitamin A.

A recent study[28] in which more than 800 patients with lacerations or surgical incisions were followed for 3 months found that suboptimal wound appearance was increased with extremity wounds, wide wounds, incompletely apposed wounds, associated tissue trauma, use of electrocautery, and infection.[28] The type of closure device and the use of deep sutures had no effect on infection rates or cosmetic appearance.

Scarring also depends on the static and dynamic tensions to which the wound is subjected. Static tensions are forces that stretch the skin over the underlying skeleton when the subject is motionless. Dynamic skin tensions are the result of forces associated with motion of joints or the face. These forces vary considerably between different individuals and between different anatomical locations. **In general, although lacerations that run parallel to the lines of minimal tension and perpendicular to underlying muscles (Fig. 1–3) usually heal with fine scars, those that are perpendicular to the lines of minimal tension often heal with wide, unsightly scars.** These scars may be revised (e.g., by performing Z-plasty) at least 6 to 12 months after injury.

A study by Wray[29] clearly demonstrated that scar width was directly related to the force required for wound closure. Methods that are designed to reduce

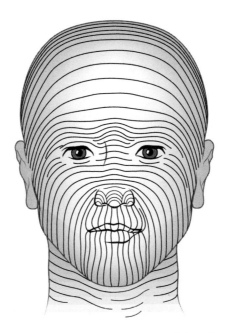

FIG. 1–3. Lines of minimal tension. Lacerations parallel to these lines will be under less tension than lacerations perpendicular to these lines and will have narrower scars.

wound tension, including wound undermining and use of deep sutures, are reviewed in Chapter 11. **The tension to which the laceration is subjected can be roughly estimated clinically by the degree of wound gaping at rest and during motion.**

REFERENCES

1. Clark, RAF (ed): The Molecular and Cellular Biology of Wound Repair, ed 2. Plenum Press, New York, 1996.
2. Singer, AJ, and Clark, RAF. Cutaneous wound healing. N Engl J Med 341:738–746, 1999.
3. Heldin, C-H, and Westermark, B: Role of platelet-derived growth factor in vivo. In Clark, RAF (ed): The Molecular and Cellular Biology of Wound Repair. Plenum Press, New York, 1996, pp 249–273.
4. Brown, EJ: Phagocytosis. Bioassays 17:109–117, 1995.
5. Rappolee, DA, Mark, D, Banda, MJ, et al: Wound macrophages express TGF-α and other growth factors in vivo: Analysis by mRNA phenotyping. Science 241:708–712, 1988.
6. Riches, DWH: Macrophage involvement in wound repair, remodeling and fibrosis. In Clark, RAF (ed): The Molecular and Cellular Biology of Wound Repair. Plenum Press, New York, 1996, pp 95–141.
7. Nanney, LB, and King, LE: Epidermal growth factor and transforming growth factor-α. In Clark, RAF (ed): The Molecular and Cellular Biology of Wound Repair. Plenum Press, New York, 1996, pp 171–194.
8. Werner, S, Smola, H, Liao, X, et al: The function of KGF in morphogenesis of epithelium and reepithelialization of wounds. Science 266:819–822, 1994.
9. Larjava, H, Salo, T, Haapasalmi, K, et al: Expression of integrins and basement membrane components by wound keratinocytes. J Clin Invest 92:1425–1435, 1993.
10. Clark, RAF, Ashcroft, GS, Spencer M-J, et al: Reepithelialization of normal human excisional wounds is associated with a switch from αvβ5 to αvβ6 integrins. Br J Dermatol 135:46–51, 1996.
11. Pilcher, BK, Dumin, JA, Sudbeck, BD, et al: Collagenase-1 is required for keratinocyte migration on a type I collagen matrix. J Cell Biol 137:1445–1457, 1997.
12. Hunt, TK: Wound Healing and Wound Infection: Theory and Surgical Practice. Appleton-Century-Crofts, New York, 1980.
13. Clark, RAF, Lanigan, JM, DellaPelle, P, et al: Fibronectin and fibrin(ogen) provide a provisional matrix for epidermal cell migration during wound reepithelialization. J Invest Dermatol 79:264–269, 1982.
14. Clark, RAF, Nielsen, LD, Welch, MP, et al: Collagen matrices attenuate the collagen synthetic response of cultured fibroblasts to TGF-β. J Cell Sci 108:1251–1261, 1995.
15. Welch, MP, Odland, GF, and Clark, RAF: Temporal relationships of F-actin bundle formation, collagen and fibronectin matrix assembly, and fibronectin receptor expression to wound contraction. J Cell Biol 110:133–145, 1990.
16. Desmouliere, A, Redar, M, et al: Apoptosis mediates the decrease in cellularity during the transition between granulation tissue and scar. Am J Path 146:56–66, 1995.
17. Folkman, J, and D'Amore, PA: Blood vessel formation: What is its molecular basis? Cell 87:1153–1155, 1996.
18. Risau, W: Mechanisms of angiogenesis. Nature 386:671–674, 1997.
19. Detmar, M, Brown, LF, Berse, B, et al: Hypoxia regulates the expression of vascular permeability factor/vascular endothelial growth factor (VPF/VEGF) and its receptors in human skin. J Invest Dermatol 108:263–268, 1997.
20. Pintucci, G, Bikfalvi, A, Klein, S, et al: Angiogenesis and the fibrinolytic system. Semin Thromb Hemost 22:517–524, 1996.
21. Iruela-Arispe, ML, and Dvorak, HF: Angiogenesis: A dynamic balance of stimulators and inhibitors. Thrombosis Haemostasis 78:672–677, 1997.
22. Desmouliere, A, and Gabbiani, G: The role of myofibroblasts in wound healing and fibrocontractive diseases. In Clark, RAF (ed): The Molecular and Cellular Biology of Wound Repair, ed. 2. Plenum Press, New York, 391–423, 1996.

23. Montesano, R, and Orci, L: Transforming growth factor-β stimulates collagen-matrix contraction by fibroblasts: Implications for wound healing. Proc Natl Acad Sci USA 85:4894–4897, 1988.
24. Clark, RAF, Folkvord, JM, Hart, CE, et al: Platelet isoforms of platelet-derived growth factor stimulate fibroblasts to contract collagen matrices. J Clin Invest 84:1036–1140, 1989.
25. Schiro, JA, Chan, BMC, Roswit, WR, et al: Integrin α2β1 (VLA-2) mediates reorganization and contraction of collagen matrices by human cells. Cell 67:403–410, 1991.
26. Madlener, M, Parks, WC, and Werner, S: Matrix metalloproteinases (MMPs) and their physiological inhibitors (TIMPs) are differentially expressed during excisional skin wound repair. Exp Cell Res 242:201–210, 1998.
27. Levenson, SM, Geever, EF, Crowley, LV, et al: The healing of rat skin wounds. Ann Surg 161:293–308, 1965.
28. Singer, AJ, Quinn, JV, Thode, HC Jr., et al: Determinants of poor outcome after laceration and surgical incision repair. Plast Reconstr Surg, 2002 (in press).
29. Wray, CR: Force required for wound closure and scar appearance. Plast Reconstr Surg 72:380–382, 1983.

JUDD E. HOLLANDER, MD

CHAPTER

2

Patient and Wound Assessment: Basic Concepts of the Patient History and Physical Examination

Evaluation of a patient with a traumatic wound begins with an expeditious, comprehensive assessment of the patient. This initial assessment can be divided into primary and secondary surveys following Advanced Trauma Life Support Algorithms. **Before focussing attention on the laceration, be certain to exclude less obvious but more serious life-threatening injuries.**

External bleeding can usually be controlled by direct pressure over the site of bleeding. Application of a tourniquet is seldom necessary and is not recommended for routine wound care. When possible, skin flaps should be returned to their original positions before application of pressure. This prevents further vascular compromise of the injured area. Amputated extremities should be covered with moist, sterile, protective dressings; placed in waterproof bags; and then placed in a container of ice water for preservation and consideration of future reattachment.

Remove any constricting rings or other jewelry from the injured body part as soon as possible. As swelling progresses rapidly, circumferential objects can act as constricting bands with resulting distal ischemia.

Patient comfort should be a priority. In most cases, pain can be reduced by compassionate and professional evaluation of the patient. Before wound preparation, most patients need some form of anesthesia (see Chapter 4). Preparing the local anesthetic out of the patient's sight may reduce anxiety caused by their seeing a needle.

MEDICAL HISTORY

Many patients may have already attempted to cleanse or care for their wound. The clinician should inquire about any treatments or home remedies that the patient has used to manage the laceration, including solutions or cleansing agents that may have been applied.

A detailed history of any allergies to anesthetic agents or antibiotics is essential. With the increased incidence of severe reactions to latex products, one must also review any prior allergies to latex. The need for further tetanus vaccination should be determined, following the recommendations of the Centers for Disease Control and Prevention (CDC)[1] (see Chapter 17).

Proper wound management begins with taking a thorough patient history that emphasizes the various factors that can have adverse effects on wound healing. Host factors such as the extremes of age, diabetes mellitus, chronic renal failure, obesity, malnutrition, and the use of immunosuppressive medications (e.g., steroids and chemotherapeutic agents) all increase the risk of wound infection and can impair wound healing.[2] Wound healing may also be impaired by inherited or acquired connective tissue disorders such as Ehlers-Danlos syndrome, Marfan syndrome, osteogenesis imperfecta, and protein and vitamin C deficiencies.[1] The tendency of patients to form keloids should be ascertained because this may result in poor scarring. Black and Asian individuals are more prone to keloid formation.[1]

The anatomic location of the injury helps predict the likelihood of infection as well as the long-term cosmetic result. In general, the body can be divided into separate anatomic areas according to the composition of the skin microflora:

- On the body surface, upper arms, and legs, the density of the bacterial population is low.
- Moist areas of the body, such as the axillae, perineum, toe webs, and intertriginous areas harbor millions of bacteria per square centimeter.
- Exposed areas of the body may also have a bacterial density in the millions per square centimeter, but the flora there are more homogeneous.
- Organisms are normally sparse on the palms and dorsa of the hands; they are in the hundreds per square centimeter.
- Most organisms on the hands (10,000 to 100,000 per square centimeter) reside beneath the distal end of the fingernail plate or adjacent to the fingernail folds.
- The oral cavity is usually heavily contaminated with facultative species and obligate anaerobes.

Obviously, any wounds with human or animal fecal contaminants run high risks of infection, even with therapeutic intervention.

In addition to bacterial flora, anatomical variation in regional blood flow also plays a role in determining the likelihood of infection (Table 2–1). Wounds located on highly vascular areas, such as the face or scalp, are less likely to be infected than are wounds located in less vascular areas.[3] The increased vascularity of the area more than offsets the high bacterial inoculum found in the scalp. **Lacerations of the scalp and face have very low infection rates regardless of the intensity of cleansing.[4]**

TABLE 2–1. RISK OF WOUND INFECTION AS A FUNCTION OF ANATOMIC LOCATION	
Location	Risk of Infection, %
Head and neck	1–2
Upper extremity	4
Lower extremity	7

Source: Unpublished data from Stony Brook Wound Registry; provided by Dr. Judd Hollander and Dr. Adam Singer.

Identification of the mechanism of injury is essential to help identify the presence of any potential wound contaminants and foreign bodies, which can result in chronic infection and delayed healing. Visible contamination of the wound doubles the risk of infection.[5] Organic and inorganic components of soil are infection potentiating; wounds contaminated by these fractions become infected with lower doses of bacterial inoculum. The major inorganic infection-potentiating particles are the clay fractions, which are most concentrated in the subsoil rather than the topsoil. Patients whose injuries occur in swamps or excavations are at high risk of being contaminated by these fractions. Some soil contaminants, such as sand grains, are relatively innocuous. Black dirt on the surface of highways appears to have minimal chemical reactivity.

The type of forces applied at the time of injury also helps predict the likelihood of infection.[6] The most common mechanism of injury is application of a blunt force such as bumping one's head against a coffee table. Such contact crushes the skin against an underlying bone, causing the skin to split. Crush injuries, which tend to cause greater devitalization of tissue, are more susceptible to infection than are wounds that have resulted from shearing forces. Mammalian bites are a relatively infrequent cause of lacerations, but the management of bite wounds differs from that of other lacerations (see Chapter 12).

Impact injuries with low energy levels may not result in division of the skin, but they can disrupt vessels, leading to an ecchymosis. Disruption of vessels in the underlying tissue results in hematoma formation. Some hematomas spontaneously resorb. Those that become encapsulated usually require treatment to prevent permanent subcutaneous deformity. While still gelatinous, a hematoma may be treated by incision and drainage. As further liquefaction occurs, aspiration with a large-bore needle ($\geq$ 18 gauge) may be possible.

WOUND EXAMINATION AND EXPLORATION

Adequate wound examination should always be conducted under optimal lighting conditions with minimal bleeding. Cursory examination under poor lighting or when the depths of the wound are obscured by blood will ultimately result in underdetection of embedded foreign bodies and damage to important structures such as tendons, nerves, or arteries. One way to minimize the possibility of missing an injury to a vital structure is to start the wound examination with a careful neurovascular assessment of pulses, motor function, and sensation distal to the laceration. Finger tourniquets may be used to obtain a bloodless field, but they should not be used for more than 30 to 60 minutes. The use of sterile technique is addressed in Chapter 3, which discusses wound preparation.

The presence of a foreign body is associated with a threefold increase in risk of infection.[5] In fact, failure to diagnose foreign bodies is the fifth leading cause of litigation against emergency physicians. Missed tendon and nerve injuries and failure to prevent infection are other common wound-related causes of litigation.

PREDICTING THE COSMETIC OUTCOME

Patients should be educated regarding their expected cosmetic outcome. They should be explicitly told that they will have some scarring. The maximal width of the scar can often be predicted based on wound location and alignment with lines of minimal tension. As discussed in Chapter 1, the location of the wound contributes to the cosmetic appearance of the scar by affecting static and dynamic skin tensions. Lacerations over joints are subject to large dynamic skin tensions and result in wider scars than similar lacerations subject to less tension. Wounds that run perpendicular to the lines of minimal skin tension are also prone to the development of wider scars (see Fig. 1–3). Patients should be educated about the expected outcome before wound closure to reduce the likelihood that the result will not meet their expectations. They should clearly understand that all traumatic lacerations result in some scarring.

REFERENCES

1. Singer, AJ, Hollander, JE, and Quinn, JV: Evaluation and management of traumatic lacerations. N Engl J Med 337:1142–1148, 1997.
2. Cruse, PJE, and Foord, R: A five-year prospective study of 23,649 surgical wounds. Arch Surg 107:206–209, 1973.
3. Hollander, JE, Singer, AJ, Valentine, S, et al: Wound registry: Development and validation. Ann Emerg Med 25:675–685, 1995.
4. Hollander, JE, Richman, PB, Werblud, M, et al: Irrigation in facial and scalp lacerations: Does it alter outcome? Ann Emerg Med 31:73–77, 1998.
5. Hollander, JE, Singer, AJ, Valentine, SM, et al: Risk factors for infection in patients with traumatic lacerations. Acad Emerg Med 8:716–720, 2001.
6. Cardany, CR, Rodeheaver, G, Thacker, J, et al: The crush injury: A high risk wound. JACEP 5:965–970, 1976.

ADAM J. SINGER, MD
JUDD E. HOLLANDER, MD

CHAPTER

3

Wound Preparation

Adequate wound preparation is one of the cornerstones of wound management. Many novice practitioners overemphasize wound closure and neglect the critical stage of wound preparation. A recent study[1] on hand lacerations suggests that many small, simple wounds can be managed conservatively without the need for closure. Properly prepared wounds often heal well without any closure at all. The purpose of wound preparation is to remove any contaminated, foreign, or devitalized tissue. It is also intended to reduce bacterial levels to a minimum in order to lessen the likelihood of wound infection and impaired healing, thus helping to attain a functional and aesthetically appealing scar, the ultimate goal of wound management.

USE OF ASEPTIC TECHNIQUE

The introduction of aseptic technique by Lister was one of the most significant advances of modern medicine, significantly reducing morbidity and mortality. Since then, the use of sterile surgical gloves, masks, and caps has become the routine procedure in surgery. Although epidemiologic studies suggest that scalp hair is a significant source of wound contamination, no reported studies have specifically demonstrated the efficacy of the practitioner's wearing a cap during wound repair in emergency or outpatient settings. Similarly, the major function of a surgical mask is to reduce contamination of the wound from saliva and nasal secretions, both of which contain large amounts of bacteria. However, a study[2] comparing 239 patients whose lacerations were repaired by a gloved operator wearing a mask and cap with 203 patients whose wounds were closed by a gloved operator without a cap or mask failed to demonstrate any differences in wound infection rates. A study by Whorl and colleagues[3] also did not identify any beneficial effects of sterile technique on wound infection rates after laceration repair. Nevertheless, the benefits of adherence to aseptic technique certainly outweigh their risks and is therefore recommended.

A mask also protects against spraying of bodily fluids from wounds into the practitioner's mouth and nose. Eye protection is also recommended to reduce the risk of transmission of bloodborne diseases.

Powdered gloves contain a variety of lubricants such as talc, cornstarch, and calcium carbonate. All of these lubricants are associated with complications such as foreign body reactions, granulomas, chronic sinus tracts, and adhesions.[4–6] The presence of these foreign materials may also increase the likelihood of infection.[6,7] As a result, many hospitals are now using powder-free gloves. With the increase in the number and severity of allergic reactions resulting from contact with latex allergens,[8,9] only latex-free gloves should be used. Wearing two pairs of surgical gloves has been shown to reduce the risk of contamination with bodily fluids during surgery.[10–12] Double gloving does require some getting used to, but it does not impair manual dexterity.[13] The use of double gloving in the emergency and outpatient settings has not been studied.

HAIR REMOVAL

Hair removal is not a prerequisite to optimal wound closure, but it does make wound closure easier. Hair can become caught within the wound or get entangled with the suture material. The hair follicles are also a significant source of bacterial contamination. Ideally, hair should be removed without traumatizing the follicles because traumatizing them may introduce bacteria into the wound and surrounding skin. Often the hair can be removed by clipping it around the wound edges with scissors. Alternatively, applying a sterile lubricant or ointment (such as Bacitracin) keeps hair out of the wound. Hair clippers with a disposable sterile head may be used if available. Shaving the hair should be avoided because it has been shown to increase wound infection rates compared with hair clipping.[14]

Before removing any hair, remember that hair provides an important landmark for precise reapproximation of the divided wound edges, particularly in the eyebrows. Removal of eyebrow hair may also result in permanent loss of hair or abnormal growth. Consequently, *hair removal of the eyebrows should be avoided.*

SKIN ANTISEPSIS

Disinfection of the skin around the wound should be initiated without contacting the wound itself. Two groups of antiseptic agents, containing either an iodophor or chlorhexidine, exhibit activity against a broad spectrum of organisms and suppress bacterial proliferation. The superiority of one antiseptic agent over another has not been demonstrated. Although these agents can reduce the bacterial concentration on intact skin, they also appear to damage the wound's defenses and invite the development of infection within the wound itself. Consequently, inadvertent spillage of these agents into the wound should be avoided. To avoid bringing contaminated material back into the wound and to minimize inadvertent spillage of the antiseptic agent, dry gauze should be soaked in the antiseptic solution and used to scrub the wound from the wound edges outward in a circular fashion.

HEMOSTASIS

During injury, blood vessels are lacerated. The magnitude of blood loss is directly related to the size of the divided vessels. Most bleeding can be stopped by applying direct pressure to the involved vessels with saline-soaked gauze and by elevating the injured limb. In many instances, bleeding can be controlled by suturing the wound. Rubbing or abrading the wound should be avoided because it dislodges thrombi and may cause further bleeding. At times, application of a sponge or gauze soaked in a vasoconstrictor solution (such as epinephrine 1:1000 or LET [a combination of lidocaine 2%, epinephrine 1:1000, and tetracaine 2%]) can help to achieve hemostasis. Persistent bleeding from small vessels should be stopped using bipolar electrosurgical coagulation. Bipolar coagulation results in less tissue damage than monopolar coagulation.[15] The use of electrocautery of any kind should be kept to a minimum, however, because it is associated with increased infection rates and suboptimal scar appearance.[16] Bleeding from the cut ends of vessels whose diameter is larger than 2 mm should be stopped with a suture ligature using a nonreactive, synthetic, absorbable suture (see Chapter 10). The divided end of the vessel should be isolated over a short length and clamped with a small, curved hemostat (Fig. 3–1). This technique is preferred over clamping the retracted vessel along with contiguous bloodstained tissue. The divided vessel ends are then ligated with sutures (Fig. 3–2). Removal of large blood clots and any hematomas helps reduce the incidence of infection.

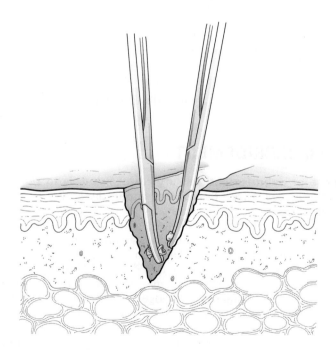

FIG. 3–1. Hemostasis is obtained by clamping the isolated bleeding vessel with a curved hemostat.

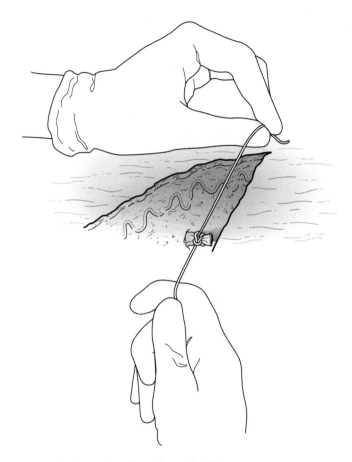

FIG. 3–2. The divided vessel ends are ligated with sutures.

SURGICAL DÉBRIDEMENT

The purpose of débridement, or surgical excision, is to remove heavily contaminated or devitalized tissues that impair the body's resistance to infection.[17] Débridement is an important element of managing some wounds, especially heavily contaminated or devitalized tissues. Nonviable tissue and irregular or crushed wound edges should be carefully débrided using a number 15 blade. Often the edges of the wound can be débrided by excising a small elliptical rim of tissue around the wound (Fig. 3–3). However, meticulous repair of irregular yet viable wound edges may be superior to their wide excision. Careful apposition of irregular wound edges provides a larger surface area of wound apposition than linear wound edges, increasing the tensile strength of the healing laceration during the remodeling period. The subcutaneous tissue may be débrided more generously, but aggressive removal of dermis should be avoided because it may result in excessive skin tension, requiring the use of

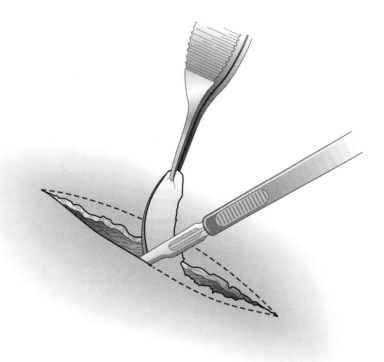

FIG. 3–3. The ragged wound edges are débrided, creating a fresh ellipsoid wound that can be approximated.

flaps or undermining to close the wound. If the margin between viable and non-viable tissue is unclear, it is better to err on the side of conservative excision. When a heavily contaminated wound contains specialized tissues such as nerves or tendons, consultation with a specialist is recommended. Generally, extensive wound débridement should only be performed in the operating room.

After wound débridement, most wounds can be closed primarily. With heavily soiled wounds, delayed primary closure (discussed later in this chapter) should be considered.

WOUND IRRIGATION

EQUIPMENT AND PROCEDURES

Wound irrigation is an effective means of removing bacteria and infection-potentiating soil fragments. Several animal wound studies[18–20] have demonstrated that the efficiency of irrigation is directly proportional to the pressure at which the fluid is delivered. These studies have also demonstrated lower infection rates for high-pressure irrigation than for low-pressure irrigation. The optimal wound irrigation pressure is not known, but studies have suggested that a pressure of at least 7 pounds per square inch (psi) may be best.[20] Whether a pulsating-jet lavage has any advantage over continuous lavage remains unclear.

In the past, a combination of a 35-mL syringe and 19-gauge needle were recommended to achieve high-pressure irrigation (> 7 psi). Recently, the forces impacted on a surface irrigated with various combinations of syringes and needles were directly measured. All combinations of syringes (10, 20, and 65 mL) and needles resulted in surface impact pressures in the range of 7 to 22 psi.[21] Replacement of the needle with a commercially available splatter shield resulted in similar impact pressures. Irrigation with a 65-mL syringe is more efficient than with smaller syringes and, when combined with a splatter shield, significantly reduces the occupational risk of contamination during wound irrigation (Figure 3–4).[22] **In general, high-pressure irrigation using a 35- or 65-mL syringe and splatter shield is advised for contaminated wounds.** Use of a basin to collect the irrigant fluid is also recommended.

The choice of the type of fluid used to irrigate wounds is more straightforward. **Although many irrigants have been tested, normal saline remains the most cost-effective and readily available choice.**[23] Because of their toxicity to healthy tissues, detergents, hydrogen peroxide, and concentrated forms of povidine iodine should not be used to irrigate wounds.[24,25]

The volume of irrigant to be used should be determined by the wound characteristics (e.g., etiology, location, time from injury) as well as host factors. Contaminated wounds with a high risk of infection require copious irrigation.

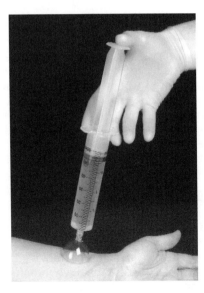

FIG. 3–4. Irrigation of a wound with a 65-mL syringe and splatter shield. The shield shown is a Zerowet Splashield (Zerowet, Inc., Palos Verdes Peninsula, Calif.).

A common recommendation, although not evidence based, is to use approximately 50 to 100 mL of irrigant per cm of wound length.

A NOTE OF CAUTION

There have been some theoretical objections to the use of high-pressure irrigation in the cleansing of traumatic wounds, with some evidence on both sides. Bhaskar and associates[18] demonstrated that the incidence of bacteremia after high-pressure lavage in a contaminated animal wound model was negligible. Fears that high-pressure irrigation would disseminate bacteria into adjacent tissue areas were also unfounded.[26] However, lateral spread of the irrigation fluid occurred in the loose areolar tissue, contributing to the development of postoperative edema. In this study, the concern that high-pressure irrigation would damage tissue defenses was justified. It resulted in trauma to the wound, which made the wound more susceptible to infection.[26] This finding serves to remind practitioners that high-pressure irrigation should not be used indiscriminately and should be reserved for highly contaminated wounds.

A recent nonrandomized, observational study[27] compared wound infection rates and cosmetic appearance 1 week after repair of 1090 facial lacerations that were irrigated versus 833 that were not irrigated. The infection rate (0.9 percent) in the irrigated wounds was similar to the rate (1.4 percent) in nonirrigated wounds. In contrast, there was a trend toward better early cosmetic appearance in the nonirrigated wounds (82 percent optimal wounds) than in the irrigated wounds (76 percent). This study suggests that high-pressure irrigation may not be required for all low-risk wounds, particularly in areas with excellent vascular supply, such as the face. High-pressure irrigation is particularly recommended for contaminated wounds in areas of poor vascular supply but should be used with caution elsewhere.

SCRUBBING

A saline-soaked sponge is an effective means of removing bacteria from the surface of the wound.[28] Scrubbing also removes the proteinaceous coagulum that prevents antibacterial agents from reaching the wound. Cleansing with a saline-soaked sponge can also significantly damage the tissue, however, impairing the wound's ability to resist infection. Sponges with a low porosity are more abrasive and inflict more damage on the tissues than do highly porous sponges. Adding a nontoxic surfactant (e.g., a surgical wound cleansing solution containing a 20% concentration of Pluronic F-68) to the sponge minimizes the tissue damage while maintaining the bacteria removal efficiency of scrubbing.[29] **Wound scrubbing is best reserved for highly contaminated wounds such as so-called "road rash," in which surface particles become embedded within the wound.**

Removal of embedded foreign particles is painful for the patient and requires either local or regional anesthesia. With some patients, scrubbing can be initiated after application of a topical anesthetic. When possible, the patient or guardian is encouraged to perform wound scrubbing for at least 5 to 10 minutes. When embedded particles remain in the wound despite initial wound cleansing, the patient may need to undergo more thorough cleansing performed in the operating room.

DRAINS

Drainage evacuates potentially harmful collections of fluids, such as pus and blood, from wounds. If there is no definite, localized fluid collection, however, drainage is prophylactic and its potentially harmful effects become more important. Drains act as retrograde conduits through which skin contaminants can gain entrance into the wound. Placement of drains within experimental wounds exposed to subinfective inoculations of bacteria greatly enhanced the rate of infection compared with undrained controls.[30] Limited data suggest that both Silastic and Penrose drains dramatically increase the infection rate of soft tissue wounds. The rate of infection when the drain was brought out through the wound was similar to the rate when the drain lay entirely within the wound, suggesting a deleterious effect of the drain per se.[30]

DELAYED PRIMARY CLOSURE

Most traumatic lacerations can be safely closed after careful and meticulous preparation. **Grossly contaminated wounds that have a high risk of infection should not be closed during the initial evaluation.** An example of such a wound is one resulting from a high-velocity gunshot or one that is grossly contaminated with feces, saliva, purulent exudates, or soil. Many such wounds can be safely closed after 4 days (i.e., delayed primary closure) if they do not become infected.[31] The effectiveness of delayed primary closure in reducing the rate of wound infections has been well established in the military context.[32]

Wounds managed by delayed primary closure should be loosely packed with sterile gauze and the patient should be closely watched. When the wound is clean and free of devitalized tissue, its edges may be approximated with minimal risk of infection.

SUMMARY OF PROCEDURES

Wound preparation should begin with hair removal, when necessary, using an electric clipper with a disposable clipper head or scissors. Removal of bacteria and dirt from the wound can be achieved by two different techniques: (1) irrigation at pressures of 7 to 20 psi, achieved by using a 35-mL or 65-mL syringe with a 19-gauge needle or splatter shield or (2) fine-pore sponges or gauze soaked in saline. Heavily contaminated wounds (e.g., with saliva, feces, or dirt) should be subject to open wound management with complementary antibiotic prophylaxis. Débridement should always be considered for heavily contaminated wounds. The use of drains potentiates rather than prevents infection. Tetanus prophylaxis should be considered for all wounds.

REFERENCES

1. Quinn, JV, Cummings, SR, Callaham, ML, et al: Suture vs. conservative management of hand lacerations (abstract). Acad Emerg Med 8:414–415, 2001.
2. Ruthman, JC, Hendricksen, D, Miller, RF, et al: Effect of cap and mask on infection rates. Ill Med J 165:397–399, 1984.
3. Whorl, GJ: Repairing skin lacerations. Can Fam Physician 33:1185–1187, 1987.
4. Ellis, H: The hazards of surgical glove dusting powders. Surg Gynecol Obstet 171:521–527, 1990.
5. McCormick, EJ: Postoperative peritoneal granulomatous inflammation caused by magnesium silicate. JAMA 116:817–821, 1941.
6. Jaffray, DC, Nade, S: Does surgical glove powder decrease the inoculum of bacteria required to produce an abscess? J R Coll Surg Edin 28:219–222, 1983.
7. Odum, BC, O'Keefe, JS, Lara, W, et al: Influence of absorbable dusting powders on wound infection. J Emerg Med 16:875–879, 1998.
8. Morales, C, Basomba, A, Carreira, J, et al: Anaphylaxis produced by rubber glove contact. Case reports and immunological identification of the antigens involved. Clin Exp Allergy 19:425–430, 1989.
9. Sussman, GL, Tarlo, S, and Dolovich, J: The spectrum of IgE-mediated responses to latex. JAMA 265:2844–2847, 1991.
10. McCue, SF, Berg, EW, and Saunders, EA. Efficacy of double-gloving as a barrier to microbial contamination during total joint arthroplasty. J Bone Joint Surg [Am] 63:811–813, 1981.
11. Matta, H, Thompson, AM, and Rainey, JB: Does wearing two pairs of gloves protect operating theatre staff from skin contamination? Br Med J 297:597–598, 1988.
12. Cohn, GM, and Seifer, DB: Blood exposure in single versus double gloving during pelvic surgery. Am J Obstet Gynecol 162:715–717, 1990.
13. Webb, JM, and Pentlow, BD: Double gloving and surgical technique. Ann R Coll Surg Engl 75:291–292, 1993.
14. Seropian, R, and Reynolds, BM: Wound infections after preoperative depilatory versus razor preparation. Am J Surg 121:251–254, 1971.
15. Ferguson, DJ: Advances in the management of surgical wounds. Surg Clin North Am 51:49–59, 1971.
16. Singer, AJ, Quinn, J, Thode, HC Jr., et al: Determinants of poor outcome after laceration and incision repair. Plast Reconstr Surg, 2002, in press.
17. Haury, B, Rodeheaver, G, Vensko, J, et al: Debridement: An essential component of traumatic wound care. Am J Surg 135:238–242, 1978.
18. Bhaskar, SN, Cutright, DE, Gross, A, et al: Water jet devices in dental practice. J Periodontol 42:658–664, 1971.
19. Madden, J ER, Schauerhamer, R, Prusak, M, et al: Applications of principles of fluid dynamics to surgical wound irrigation. Curr Topics Surg Res 3:85–93, 1971.
20. Stevenson, TR, Thacker, JG, Rodeheaver, GT, et al: Cleansing the traumatic wound with high pressure syringe irrigation. JACEP 5:17–21, 1976.
21. Singer, AJ, and Mittra, E: Comparison of wound irrigation impact pressures (abstract). Acad Emerg Med 6:469, 1999.
22. Pigman, EC, Karch, DB, and Scott, JL: Splatter during jet irrigation cleansing of a wound model: A comparison of three inexpensive devices. Ann Emerg Med 22:1563–1567, 1993.
23. Dire, DJ, and Welsh, AP: A comparison of wound irrigation solutions used in the emergency department. Ann Emerg Med 19:704–708, 1990.
24. Fadis, D, Daniel, D, and Boyer, J: Tissue toxicity of antiseptic solutions: A study of rabbit articular and periarticular tissues. J Trauma 17:895–897, 1977.
25. Oberg, MS, and Lindsey, D. Do not put hydrogen peroxide or povidine iodine into wounds. J Trauma 20:323–324, 1980.
26. Wheeler, CB, Rodeheaver, GT, Thacker, JG, et al: Side-effects of high pressure irrigation. Surg Gynecol Obstet 143:775–778, 1976.
27. Hollander, JE, Richman, PB, Werblud, M, et al: Irrigation in facial and scalp lacerations: Does it alter outcome? Ann Emerg Med 31:73–77, 1998.
28. Rodeheaver, GT, Smith, SL, Thacker, JG, et al: Mechanical cleansing of contaminated wounds with a surfactant. Am J Surg 129:241–245, 1975.

29. Rodeheaver, GT, Kurtz, L, Kircher, BJ, et al: Pluronic F-68: A promising new skin wound cleanser. Ann Emerg Med 9:572–576, 1980.

30. Magee, C, Rodeheaver, GT, Golden, GT, et al: Potentiation of wound infection by surgical drains. Am J Surg 131:547–549, 1976.

31. Edlich, RF, Rogers, W, Kasper, G, et al: Studies in the management of the contaminated wound. I. Optimal time for closure of contaminated open wounds. II. Comparison of resistance to infection of open and closed wounds during healing. Am J Surg 117:323–329, 1969.

32. Heaton, LD, Hughes, CW, Rosegay, H, et al: Military surgical practices of the United States Army in Vietnam. Curr Probl Surg 1–59, 1966.

JOEL M. BARTFIELD, MD

Wound Anesthesia

Patients who have suffered even minor wounds may be emotionally traumatized and anxious when presenting to the emergency department for care. Maintaining a calming, supportive environment helps to ensure patient cooperation during wound treatment. It is important to take a few minutes to allay patients' anxiety and address their concerns. Even the most stoic-appearing patients may be concerned about the pain associated with injection of anesthesia; therefore, it is important to take steps to minimize pain associated with anesthesia administration. One study[1], for example, found that patients who listened to music during laceration repair reported less pain and anxiety than those who did not. Although it may not be possible to provide music for patients in many emergency settings, physicians should make every effort to minimize patient anxiety during wound care. For example, withdrawing anesthetic agents and preparing needles and syringes should be done out of the view of patients.

METHODS OF ANESTHETIC ADMINISTRATION: LOCAL VERSUS REGIONAL ANESTHESIA

Proper wound evaluation and management often require anesthesia. For many wounds, anesthesia is accomplished through local infiltration of anesthetic agents directly into the wound. This technique has several advantages. It is easy to accomplish, and it is reliable and safe as long as proper techniques are used and toxicity is not exceeded. Additionally, local infiltration, particularly with anesthetic agents that contain epinephrine, provides local hemostasis.

However, local anesthesia also has several noteworthy disadvantages. Infiltration of anesthetic agents in and around wounds distorts anatomy and can make subsequent repair of lacerations more difficult. It also often requires multiple injections. Table 4–1 summarizes the advantages and disadvantages of local anesthetic agents, topical anesthetic agents, and nerve blocks.

TABLE 4–1. COMPARISON OF TYPES OF ANESTHESIA

Type	Advantages	Disadvantages
Local	Ease of technique	May require high volumes of anesthetic agent
	Reliability	May be excessively painful in certain locations (e.g., tips of extremities, palms, soles)
		Distorts anatomy, possibly impeding optimal wound edge approximation
Topical	Painless	Not always reliable (works best on face)
	Does not distort anatomy	Danger of absorption if used on mucous membranes
		Cannot be used on areas with end-arteriolar circulation
Nerve or field blocks	Does not distort anatomy	Only useful for certain locations
	Requires lower volume of anesthetic	Not as reliable as local anesthesia
	Fewer injections	

LOCAL ANESTHESIA

REDUCING THE PAIN OF INFILTRATION

Although local infiltration of anesthetic agents is effective and reliable, it is also associated with significant pain and anxiety. Several techniques can be incorporated to minimize the pain of anesthetic infiltration. Factors shown to influence the pain of anesthetic infiltration include the type of anesthetic,[2] needle size,[3] pH[4] and temperature of the solution,[5] and speed and depth of injection.[6] **Therefore, steps to minimize the pain of infiltration of local anesthetic agents include buffering, subcutaneous rather than intradermal injection, slow rate of injection, injecting from within wound margins, and pretreating wounds with a topical anesthetic agent.**

Local anesthetic agents are weak bases that are marketed in solutions that are slightly acidic in order to increase their shelf life. Several studies[4] have shown that buffering solutions to approximately physiologic pH decreases the pain of infiltration. This may be the result of increasing the ratio of uncharged to charged molecules as the pH of the solution nears the anesthetic's pKa. Only uncharged molecules are readily diffusable across cell membranes, so the onset of anesthesia is more rapid; therefore, infiltration may be less painful. Anesthetic agents can be buffered by adding a small amount of sodium bicarbonate (1 mEq/mL) in approximately a 10:1 dilution to anesthetic (i.e., 10 mL of anesthetic to 1 mL of sodium bicarbonate). This can be accomplished by adding 2 mL of sodium bicarbonate to a 20-mL vial of anesthetic agent.

Buffered lidocaine can be used for up to a week after preparation with no clinical change in efficacy.[7]

Other techniques have been used to try to reduce the pain of infiltration:

* Some studies[5] have suggested that warming solutions decreases pain of infiltration, but this method has not always been found to be effective.
* Two clinical trials[8,9] have demonstrated that pain is lessened by infiltration of local anesthetic agents from within the wound rather through intact skin.
* Slow infiltration is believed to be less painful than rapid infiltration.[3]
* Subcutaneous injection is less painful than intradermal injection.[6]

Finally, pretreating wounds with topical tetracaine reduces the pain of infiltration.[10] Pretreatment of lacerations with LET (a combination of lidocaine 2%, epinephrine 1:1000, and tetracaine 2%) reduced the pain of anesthetic injection by 50 percent over placebo.[11] Topical application of EMLA Cream (lidocaine 2.5% and prilocaine 2.5%) has also been shown to reduce the pain of injection, but it is more costly than LET.[12] **Application of a topical anesthetic at the time of patient triage is both feasible and effective in reducing the pain of injection. It also saves time because by the time the patient is evaluated by the practitioner, the wound is often numb and ready to be injected.**[11]

TOPICAL ANESTHETIC AGENTS

A number of different combinations of agents have been studied as topical anesthetic agents, which would eliminate the need for needle infiltration. The combination that has been studied and used most extensively is TAC (a combination of tetracaine 0.5 %, adrenaline 1:2000, and cocaine 11.8%). However, TAC is inferior to lidocaine infiltration on wounds other than those involving the face and scalp.[13] TAC is also less effective for large lacerations,[13] and it needs to be left in place for at least 10 to 15 minutes in order to achieve anesthesia. Because of its vasoconstrictive properties, TAC is contraindicated on areas supplied by end arterioles. It cannot be used on mucous membrane abrasions and burns because of enhanced cocaine absorption.[13] Inappropriate use of TAC on mucous membranes has been associated with seizures and death.[14,15]

Local anesthesia can be provided without infiltration through combination topical anesthetic agents. Topical 5% lidocaine with epinephrine and LET have both compared favorably with TAC.[16] The major advantages of LET over TAC are its improved safety profile and lack of administrative problems associated with using controlled substances.

EMLA Cream, a eutectic mixture of lidocaine and prilocaine, has been used successfully as an anesthetic agent on intact skin before invasive procedures such as phlebotomy, intravenous (IV) catheter insertion, and lumbar puncture.[17] The agent is not currently approved by the Food and Drug Administration (FDA) for use on non-intact skin, but a recent study[18] found EMLA Cream to be superior to TAC for anesthesia of simple extremity lacerations.

Approximately 1 hour was required before optimal anesthesia was achieved. Therefore, LET is recommended due to its low cost. Singer and Stark[12] found no differences in the anesthetic efficacies of EMLA Cream and LET before injection of lacerations with lidocaine.

JET INJECTION AND IONTOPHORESIS

Traditional local anesthetic agents can be "infiltrated" into skin without the use of a needle. Two techniques that have been shown to be effective for this purpose are jet injection and iontophoresis.

Jet injection involves the use of a device that essentially sprays material into skin at high pressure (200 pounds per square inch [psi]). Small amounts (0.1 mL) of anesthetic can be infiltrated in this way to a depth of 1.5 cm. The technique is limited by the fact that only small amounts of the agent can be delivered at a time.[19] Jet injection is not widely available.

Iontophoresis takes advantage of the fact that anesthetic agents exist in solution as salts of weak bases and therefore are positively charged. They can be forced into the skin by being exposed to an electric field in which the positively charged anesthetic agent is repelled by the positive pole. This technique has been shown to be effective in delivering anesthetic agents in volunteer subjects and is an effective method of providing local anesthesia before IV catheter placement.[20] The technique has not been studied as a means of providing anesthesia for lacerations. Widespread use of iontophoresis is limited by the fact that it requires special equipment and several minutes to deliver anesthetic agents. Furthermore, its application is associated with a stinging, electric shock-like sensation that may not be acceptable to many patients, especially children.

REGIONAL ANESTHESIA

FIELD BLOCKS

Field blocks involve infiltration of an anesthetic agent, either surrounding an area or interrupting the nerve supply to that area. Field blocks can only be used in certain areas of the body with appropriate sensory innervation, such as the forehead, forearm, ear, and nose. They can provide reliable anesthesia without disrupting anatomy, facilitating accurate wound edge approximation in cosmetically important areas.

NERVE BLOCKS

Several areas of the body can be anesthetized by nerve blocks (Table 4–2). **Nerve blocks usually require a smaller volume of anesthetic than does local infiltration. Additionally, nerve blocks do not distort anatomy and can often be accomplished with a single injection.** Knowledge of anatomy is critical for successfully performing nerve blocks. Care should be taken to identify landmarks. Patients may feel paresthesias during the technique. (In fact,

TABLE 4–2. LOCATIONS AMENABLE TO REGIONAL BLOCKS	
Location of Laceration	**Regional Nerve Block**
Forehead	Supraorbital
Upper eyelid	Supraorbital
Lower eyelid	Infraorbital
Upper lip	Infraorbital
Side of nose	Infraorbital
Lower lip	Mental
Fingers and toes	Digital
Radial palm and fingers	Median
Ulnar palm and fingers	Ulnar
Dorsum of hand	Radial
Sole of foot	Sural and tibial
Lateral aspect of foot	Sural
Dorsum of foot	Superficial and deep peroneal

paresthesias indicate that the drug is being delivered in an area very close to the nerve). If paresthesias are elicited, the needle should be withdrawn slightly and then the anesthetic agent should be injected. Because vascular structures tend to be located near many nerves, it is important to aspirate before injecting to make sure that the tip of the needle is not in an artery or vein. An adequate amount of anesthetic agent should be injected in the area of the nerve. After infiltration, the practitioner should gently massage the area to help to diffuse the agent into the nerve being blocked. It is important to realize that it may take several minutes for nerve blocks to take effect. If a block has been unsuccessful, the practitioner has the option of attempting the block again or resorting to local anesthesia, remembering not to exceed the maximum allowable amount of local anesthetic agent.

An exhaustive review of all nerve blocks is beyond the scope of this text, but this chapter does outline several of the most commonly used blocks, which are particularly useful. These include digital nerve blocks and blocks that involve nerves supplying sensation to the hands, feet, and face.

Digital Nerve Block

Digital nerve blocks are the most commonly performed nerve block. Injuries of the digits are common, and the technique of blocking digital nerves is easily learned. Two sets of digital nerves (i.e., palmar and dorsal) each run along the lateral aspect of the digit. Because the palmar nerves supply most of the sensation to the fingertips, nerve block at this location is generally all that is required. For the thumb and fifth digit, the dorsal nerves must also be blocked to provide complete anesthesia. Care must be taken to avoid injury to vascular structures when performing these blocks because blood vessels run in close proximity to digital nerves. Because digital arteries provide end arterial circulation to the finger and toe tips, anesthetic agents that contain epinephrine should be avoided in these locations.

There are several acceptable techniques for performing digital nerve blocks. The nerve can be blocked either at the metacarpophalangeal (MCP) joint or anywhere along its course. MCP blocks are performed by inserting a needle into the web space between the digits on either side of the digit being blocked and depositing the anesthetic near the joint (Fig. 4–1). This technique is relatively easy to learn. One study[21] involving 30 volunteers compared it with a block performed along the digit and found the MCP block to be less reliable (23 percent vs. 3 percent failure rate) and to have a slower onset (6.35 vs. 2.82 minutes). Conventional digital blocks can be performed by introducing the needle through the dorsal or ventral surface of the digit at its base (Fig. 4–2). Buffered lidocaine has been shown to be less painful to administer for digital nerve blocks than plain lidocaine.[22]

Nerve Blocks of the Hand

An appreciation for the sensory innervation of the hand is essential when choosing appropriate nerve blocks for hand injuries. Figure 4–3 shows the typical sensory innervation of the hand. However, innervation is variable, so more than one block may be required for wounds in certain locations. Because in-

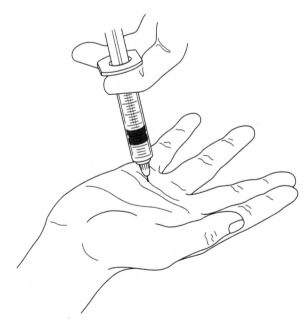

FIG. 4–1. Metacarpal block. A metacarpal block can be performed through needle insertion beneath the skin overlying the distal palmar crease. Anesthesia is then injected on either side of the metacarpal joint.

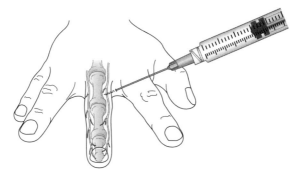

FIG. 4–2. Digital nerve blocks. A digital block can be performed with injection of anesthesia either along the sides of the digit just distal to the web space or into the web space on either side of the digit to be anesthetized.

filtration of local anesthetic agents into the hand (particularly into the thick palmar skin) can be especially painful, practitioners should learn how to use these blocks when clinically indicated.

Ulnar Nerve Block. The ulnar nerve can be blocked at the wrist or the elbow, but the wrist is the preferable location. At the elbow, the nerve can easily be damaged because of its superficial location and close proximity to bony structures. At the wrist, the ulnar nerve lies between the flexor carpi ulnaris tendon

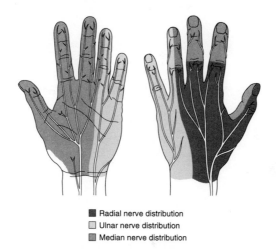

■ Radial nerve distribution
□ Ulnar nerve distribution
■ Median nerve distribution

FIG. 4–3. Sensory innervation of the hand. In most patients the ulnar nerve provides sensation to both the palmar and dorsal surfaces of the 5th digit and ulnar half of the 4th digit. The median nerve provides sensation to the first three digits and the radial aspect of the 4th digit on the palmar side. The radial nerve provides sensory innervation to the first 3½ digits of the dorsal surface of the hand and proximal phalanx. Innervation to the skin overlying the middle and distal phalanges of the first 3½ digits has a contribution from the median nerve, as well as the radial nerve.

and the ulnar artery (Fig. 4–4A). The nerve can be blocked either by introducing the needle between these two structures or, preferably, by introducing the needle underneath the flexor carpi ulnaris tendon at the ulnar aspect of the wrist. With either technique, care should be taken to avoid injection into the ulnar artery by aspirating before injection. A total of 5 to 7 mL of agent is injected to achieve anesthesia.

Median Nerve Block. The median nerve is located between the palmaris longus and the flexor carpi radialis tendons. The palmaris longus tendon can be located by having the patient oppose the thumb and fifth finger and flex the wrist against resistance. This tendon is congenitally absent approximately 20 percent the time. In these instances, the nerve can be found approximately 1 cm ulnar to the flexor carpi radialis. The median nerve is blocked by puncturing the flexor retinaculum between the two wrist creases at the location of the nerve and injecting 5 to 8 mL of agent at this site (See Fig. 4–5A).

Radial Nerve Block. The radial nerve follows the radial artery and then fans out dorsally distal to the wrist. The nerve is blocked by injecting into the anatomic snuff box and laying a 6- to 8-cm wheal of anesthetic agent as a field block across the dorsal portion of the radial aspect of the wrist (Fig. 4–5B).

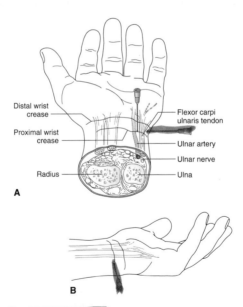

Distal wrist crease
Proximal wrist crease
Radius
Flexor carpi ulnaris tendon
Ulnar artery
Ulnar nerve
Ulna

A

B

FIG. 4–4A AND B. *Ulnar nerve block.* The ulnar nerve lies just radial to the flexor carpi ulnaris tendon, which can be best identified at the wrist creases when the wrist is in forced flexion and ulnar deviation. The palmar branch can be anesthetized through injection just radial to the flexor carpi ulnaris tendon at the proximal wrist crease. To anesthetize the dorsal branch, a subcutaneous wheal should be placed, extending from over the flexor carpi ulnaris tendon around the ulnar side of the wrist to the middle of the dorsal aspect of the wrist.

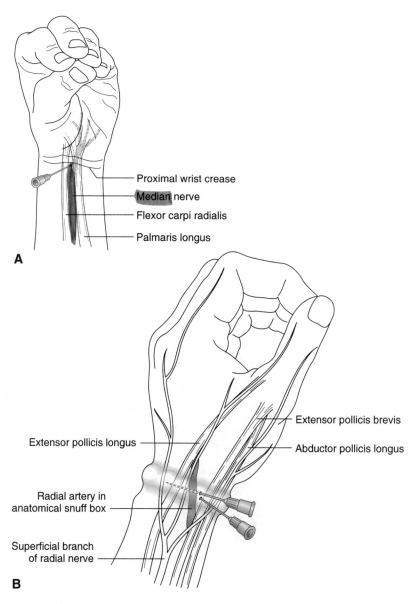

FIG. 4–5A. Median nerve block. Having the patient make a fist and flex the wrist against resistance can identify the landmarks for a median nerve block. At the proximal wrist crease, the nerve lies just radial to the tendon of the palmaris longus. **B. Radial nerve blocks** can be performed by injection of anesthesia into the anatomic snuff box in combination with laying a subcutaneous wheal of anesthesia across the portion of the wrist that extends dorsally from this point.

Nerve Blocks of the Foot

Nerve Blocks of the Ankle. Depending on the area of injury, anesthesia of the foot can be provided by five different nerve blocks at the ankle. Because the anatomy is somewhat variable, the nerves are often blocked in groups. The sole of the foot is supplied by the tibial nerve (which branches into the medial and lateral plantar nerve) and the sural nerve (Fig. 4–6). The most lateral aspect of the dorsum of the foot is supplied by the sural nerve, with the remainder supplied by the superficial and deep peroneal nerves and the saphenous nerve (see Fig. 4–6). Ankle blocks are somewhat more difficult to accomplish than the other blocks discussed in this chapter. Familiarity with these blocks can be very useful, however, local anesthesia to the sole of the foot is particularly difficult to accomplish and is painful to administer because of the thickness of the skin in this location.

Tibial Nerve (Medial and Lateral Plantar Nerves) Block. The tibial nerve runs between the medial malleolus and the Achilles tendon in close proxim-

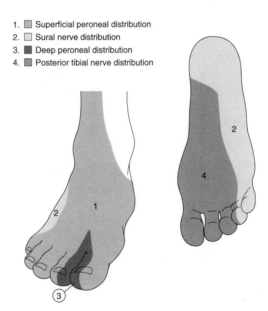

1. ▨ Superficial peroneal distribution
2. ▢ Sural nerve distribution
3. ■ Deep peroneal distribution
4. ▨ Posterior tibial nerve distribution

FIG. 4–6. Sensory innervation of the foot. The common peroneal nerve splits into a superficial and deep branch. The superficial branch supplies most of the skin on the dorsum of the foot, including all the digits except the lateral side of the 5th and the adjacent portions of the 1st and 2nd digits, as shown. The deep peroneal nerve supplies sensation to the contiguous sides of the 1st and 2nd digits. Most of the plantar sensory innervation of the foot comes from the medial plantar nerve, which supplies the medial side of the sole of the foot and the first three digits. The lateral plantar nerve provides sensation to the lateral aspect of the sole and the 4th and 5th digits. Calcaneal branches of the tibial and sural nerves supply sensation to the heel. The saphenous nerve supplies sensation to the medial side of the foot up to the first metatarsal head. The sural nerve supplies sensation to the lateral aspect of the foot.

ity to the tibia. This nerve is blocked by injecting 5 mL of anesthetic agent between the posterior tibial artery and the Achilles tendon just posterior to the medial malleolus (Fig. 4–7A). This block is best accomplished with the patient in the prone position. It can take up to 10 to 15 minutes to achieve anesthesia because of the thickness of the nerve in this location.

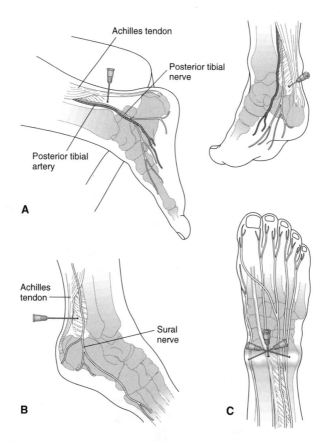

FIG. 4–7. Regional blocks around the ankle. *(A)* The posterior tibial nerve block is best identified with the patient in the prone position. Using a 2-inch-long needle, the anesthesia should be injected just medial to the Achilles tendon and lateral to the tibial artery posterior to the medial malleolus. A posterior tibial nerve block will provide anesthesia to the medial sole of the foot (the distribution of the medial plantar nerve). *(B)* The sural nerve block should be performed with injection 1 cm above the lateral malleolus between the lateral malleolus and the Achilles tendon. *(C)* The deep peroneal nerve can be blocked anteriorly 1 cm above the base of the medial malleolus. The patient should dorsiflex the great toe and foot to identify the extensor hallucis longus and anterior tibial tendons. Anesthesia can be injected 1 cm above the distal end of the tibia in 30-degree angles from the skin entrance. The superficial peroneal nerve can be blocked with an injection that extends in a line from the anterior border of the tibia to the lateral malleolus. Extension medially at the same level will block the saphenous nerve.

Sural Nerve Block. The sural nerve is located between the lateral malleolus and the Achilles tendon. The sural nerve is relatively superficial compared with the tibial nerve, so it requires a more superficial injection. The sural nerve can be blocked by injecting 5 mL of anesthetic agent superficially in a fan-like distribution just lateral to the Achilles tendon at the top of the lateral malleolus (Fig. 4–7B).

Superficial Peroneal, Deep Peroneal, and Saphenous Nerve Blocks. All three of these nerves should be blocked in order to provide adequate anesthesia to the dorsum of the foot. With the patient in a supine position, the skin is entered between lateral to the extensor hallucis longus at a point parallel to the superior aspect of the medial malleolus. The deep peroneal nerve is blocked by a deep injection between the two tendons (Fig. 4–7C). The needle is then withdrawn and redirected subcutaneously toward the lateral malleolus to block the superficial peroneal nerve and then medially to block the saphenous nerve (Fig. 4–7C). A total of 15 mL of agent is usually required to block all three nerves.

Nerve Blocks of the Face

Facial lacerations require special attention in order to achieve the best possible cosmetic result. Nerve blocks are ideal for facial lacerations because they do not distort anatomy and are relatively easy to perform. The trigeminal nerve supplies sensation to the face. The three branches of this nerve commonly blocked are the supraorbital, infraorbital, and mental nerves. All of these nerves exit from foramina that fall along a line that connects the medial aspect of the pupil with the corner of the mouth (Fig. 4–8).

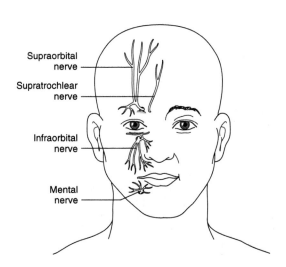

Supraorbital nerve

Supratrochlear nerve

Infraorbital nerve

Mental nerve

FIG. 4–8. Sensory innervation of the face. The supraorbital nerve supplies sensation to most of the forehead, although the supratrochlear nerve provides sensation to the most medial aspect of the forehead. The infraorbital nerve provides sensation to the skin beneath the eye, extending down to the upper lip and including the cheek. The mental nerve innervates the skin of the lower lip and the chin.

Supraorbital Nerve Block. The supraorbital nerve supplies sensation to most of the forehead; the area near the bridge of the nose is innervated by the supratrochlear nerve. The supraorbital nerve exits at the supraorbital foramen, and the supratrochlear nerve exits 5 to 10 mm medial to it (Fig. 4–9). Both nerves can be blocked at this easily identifiable location. The supraorbital nerve is blocked by directing the needle at the supraorbital foramen until it hits underlying bone, after which the anesthetic agent is injected. Raising a subcutaneous wheal of anesthetic directly above and parallel to the medial eyebrow blocks the supratrochlear branch.

Infraorbital Nerve Block. The infraorbital nerve exits through the infraorbital foramen, which is easily palpated along the line previously described, just below the inferior border of the orbit. The nerve supplies sensation to the medial aspect of the mid-face, including the upper lip. The infraorbital nerve can be blocked either by injection through intact skin or through buccal mucosa (Fig. 4–10). Injection through the mucosa involves inserting a ¾-inch needle to the hub into the buccal-mucosal sulcus opposite the upper canine and palpating the foramen as the anesthetic agent is introduced. Care must be taken to introduce the needle along the surface of the maxilla in order to avoid the globe and not penetrate the skin of the face. This intraoral technique was shown to be more reliable and less painful than the transcutaneous method of injection in a study[23] that involved 12 volunteers. However, many have discouraged its use because of the risk of a needle-stick injury. Alternatively, the

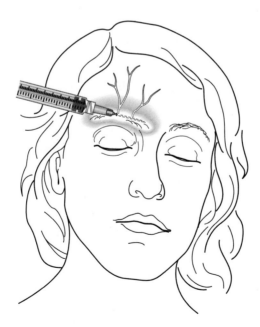

FIG. 4–9. Supraorbital nerve block. The supraorbital nerve is anesthetized at the point of origination in the superior orbital rim. A wheal of anesthesia can extend medially to block the supratrochlear nerve also.

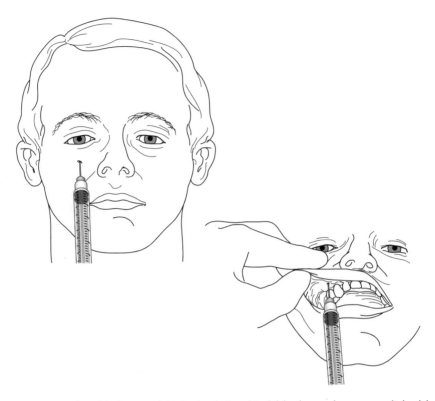

FIG. 4–10. Infraorbital nerve block. An infraorbital block can be accomplished by transcutaneous route, whereby the skin is penetrated just beneath the infraorbital notch. The intraoral approach can also be used. The injection occurs at the same location. Using either route, the practitioner should keep a gloved finger above the point of injection but beneath the patient's eye, to prevent accidental puncture of the globe.

nerve can be blocked by inserting a needle through the skin and directing it at the infraorbital foramen (see Fig. 4–10).

Mental Nerve Block. The mental nerve supplies sensation to the superior chin and lower lip. The nerve exits through the mental foramen, which can be palpated along the previously described line in the lateral chin. As with the infraorbital nerve, there are two approaches to blocking the mental nerve; they are transcutaneous or intraoral injection. The intraoral approach is accomplished by inserting a ¾-inch needle to the hub into the buccal-alveolar mucosal fold opposite the lower canine and palpating the foramen as the anesthetic is introduced (Fig. 4–11). This usually requires directing the needle laterally at a 45-degree angle. The intraoral technique was shown to be more reliable and less painful in a study[24] that involved 10 volunteers.

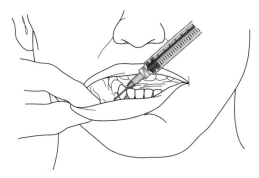

FIG. 4–11. Mental nerve block. In the intraoral approach, the needle enters the alveolar-buccal junction opposite the canine and angled downward toward the mental foramina.

CLINICAL CONSIDERATIONS OF ANESTHETIC AGENT SELECTION

Local and regional anesthetics are generally either amide or esters of the "-caine" family. Esters were the first to be developed, of which procaine (Novocain) is the prototype. Unlike amide anesthetic agents, which are metabolized by the liver, ester anesthetic agents are metabolized in plasma by pseudo-cholinesterases. Compared with amides, esters have a relatively high incidence of allergic reactions. Therefore, amides (e.g., lidocaine) are used most often.

DOSING AND TOXICITY

Local anesthetic agents have dose-related toxicities. Dosing by weight (i.e., mg/kg) is useful in pediatric patients, but the maximum safe doses in adults are generally expressed in absolute terms because weight does not correlate well with peak anesthetic drug levels in adults.[25] The maximum safe amount of plain lidocaine in an adult patient is 300 mg. A 1% solution contains 1000 mg per 100 mL, or 10 mg/mL. Therefore, the maximum amount of 1% lidocaine that can be safely used in an adult patient is 30 mL. This dose refers to subcutaneous or intradermal injections. Toxicity may occur at a much lower dose if anesthetics are inadvertently injected intravascularly. Table 4–3 provides generally accepted maximum doses for commonly used local anesthetics.

The practitioner has several choices if volumes that approach toxicity are required:

- Selection of a less toxic agent
- Dilution of the agent
- Providing anesthesia as a nerve or field block, which often requires less volume than simple local anesthesia
- The addition of epinephrine

TABLE 4–3. MAXIMUM SAFE DOSES FOR SELECTED ANESTHETICS

Generic Name	Trade Name	Classification	Adult Dose, mg	Pediatric Dose, mg/kg
Lidocaine	Xylocaine	Amide	300	4
Lidocaine with epinephrine	Xylocaine with epinephrine	Amide	500	7
Bupivacaine	Marcaine	Amide	175	1.5
Bupivacaine with epinephrine	Marcaine with epinephrine	Amide	225	3
Procaine	Novocain	Ester	500	7
Procaine with epinephrine	Novocain with epinephrine	Ester	600	9

Epinephrine at a concentration of approximately 1:100,000 can be added to anesthetic agents or is commercially available for some agents. The vasoconstrictive properties of epinephrine increase the amount of agent that can be safely injected by decreasing systemic absorption. They also provide a less bloody field. However, there are also several potential disadvantages to the use of epinephrine. By causing vasoconstriction, epinephrine is commonly believed to increase the risk of wound infections; however, this has not been substantiated in clinical trials. In addition, anesthetic agents that contain epinephrine have been shown to be more painful to inject.[2] **Anesthetic agents that contain epinephrine or any other vasoconstrictor should be avoided in regions of the body with end-arteriolar supply, such as the digits.**

ALLERGIES TO LOCAL ANESTHETIC AGENTS

It is common for patients to report an allergy to local anesthetic agents. True anaphylaxis to local anesthetics, particularly amides, is extremely rare.[26] Skin testing among patients with reported allergies to lidocaine has shown that very few reactions represent true allergies. Nonetheless, anaphylaxis is a potentially lethal complication that is obviously best avoided.

The first step in evaluating a patient who states that he or she is allergic to local anesthetic agents is to try to sort out the true nature of the previous reaction. Patients are often unable to distinguish a true allergic reaction from a vasovagal reaction. Anesthetics from an alternate class (e.g., amide or ester) could be used if the specific allergen was known.

The situation is further complicated by the fact that patients who report a true allergy to lidocaine are most often allergic to methylparaben, the preservative used in multidose vials, rather than to lidocaine itself. The traditional alternatives to the amide anesthetics (e.g., lidocaine, bupivicaine, mepivacaine) are the ester anesthetics (e.g., procaine, tetracaine), whose degradation product is para-amino benzoic acid (PABA), a chemical that is closely related to methylparaben and could possibly induce the same allergic reaction. If one knew with certainty that a given patient was allergic to methylparaben rather than to lidocaine itself, a reasonable alternative would be to use single-dose lidocaine (i.e., cardiac preparations of lidocaine), which contains no preservatives. However, it is difficult for physicians and patients alike to make this distinction. Therefore, alternatives to traditional anesthetics have been sought.

ALTERNATIVES TO TRADITIONAL ANESTHETIC AGENTS

Alternative non-"caine" agents that are available for patients with allergies to local anesthetics include 1% diphenhydramine and 0.9% benzyl alcohol.

Diphenhydramine

Diphenhydramine (Benadryl) is an antihistamine that is a potential substitute for lidocaine.[27] The chemical structure of antihistamines is closely related to that of local anesthetics, but it is dissimilar enough that cross-reactivity is not a concern. Although it is more painful to administer, 1% diphenhydramine provides anesthesia comparable to 1% lidocaine.[27] Diluting the concentration to 0.5% or buffering is not helpful.[28] Side effects associated with diphenhydramine include sedation, local irritation, erythema, vesicle formation, tissue necrosis, and prolonged anesthesia.[27,28] Because of the relative discomfort of diphenhydramine infiltration and potential side effects, an alternative non-"caine" anesthetic would be desirable for patients who are allergic to lidocaine.

Benzyl Alcohol

Benzyl alcohol (as found as a preservative in multidose normal saline) has minimal pain of infiltration and provides good anesthesia.[29,30] Benzyl alcohol has low toxicity, even in parenteral administration.[31] Wightman and Vaughan[2] compared benzyl alcohol with five other anesthetic agents and found that benzyl alcohol was the least painful. Its use is limited by a short duration of action (i.e., only a few minutes).[2] **The duration of action of 0.9% benzyl alcohol can be extended through the addition of epinephrine 1:100,000.**[29]

In a three-way comparison[32] with 1% diphenhydramine and 0.9% buffered lidocaine, benzyl alcohol with epinephrine 1:100,000 was found to be the least painful. Benzyl alcohol with epinephrine has also been compared with lidocaine with epinephrine in patients with simple lacerations. It caused slightly less pain upon infiltration, but eight of the 26 patients who received benzyl alcohol with epinephrine needed additional anesthesia, compared with only two of 26 in the lidocaine group. Although this difference was not statistically significant, practitioners should be aware that benzyl alcohol with epinephrine may have a relatively short duration of action in the clinical setting.[32] A solution containing benzyl alcohol with epinephrine 1:100,000 can be made by adding 0.2 mL of epinephrine 1:1000 to a 20-mL vial of multidose normal saline containing 0.9% benzyl alcohol.

REFERENCES

1. Menegazzi, JJ, et al: A randomized, controlled trial of the use of music during laceration repair. Ann Emerg Med 20:348–350, 1991.
2. Wightman, MA, and Vaughan, RW: Comparison of compounds used for intradermal anesthesia. Anesthesiology 45:687–689, 1976.
3. Berk, WA, Welch, RD, and Bock, BF: Controversial issues in clinical management of the simple wound. Ann Emerg Med 21:72–80, 1992.
4. Bartfield, JM, et al: Buffered versus plain lidocaine as a local anesthetic for simple laceration repair. Ann Emerg Med 19:1387–1389, 1990.
5. Bartfield, JM, et al: The effects of warming and buffering on pain of infiltration of lidocaine. Acad Emerg Med 2:254–258, 1995.
6. Krause, RS, et al: The effect of injection speed on the pain of lidocaine infiltration. Acad Emerg Med 4:1032–1035, 1997.
7. Bartfield, JM, et al: Buffered lidocaine as a local anesthetic: An investigation of shelf life. Ann Emerg Med 21:16–19, 1992.
8. Kelly, AM, Cohen, M, and Richards, D: Minimizing the pain of local infiltration anesthesia for wounds by injection into the wound edges. J Emerg Med 12:593–595, 1994.
9. Bartfield, JM, Sokaris, SJ, and Raccio-Roback, N: Local anesthesia for lacerations: Pain of infiltration inside versus outside the wound. Acad Emerg Med, 5:100–104, 1998.
10. Bartfield, JM, et al: Topical tetracaine attenuates the pain of infiltration of buffered lidocaine. Acad Emerg Med 3:1001–1005, 1996.
11. Singer, AJ, and Stark, MJ: Feasibility of triage nurse application of topical anesthesia for lacerations. Acad Emerg Med 6:469, 1999.
12. Singer, AJ, and Stark, MJ: EMLA versus LET for pretreating lacerations. A randomized trial. Acad Emerg Med 8:223–230, 2001.
13. Hegenbarth, MA, et al: Comparison of topical tetracaine, adrenaline, and cocaine anesthesia with lidocaine infiltration for repair of lacerations in children. Ann Emerg Med 9:63–67, 1990.
14. Dailey, RH: Fatality secondary to misuse of TAC solution. Ann Emerg Med 17:159–160, 1988.
15. Daya, MR, et al: Recurrent seizures following mucosal application of TAC. Ann Emerg Med 17:646–648, 1988.
16. Ernst, AA, et al: LAT (lidocaine-adrenaline-tetracaine) versus TAC (tetracaine-adrenaline-cocaine) for topical anesthesia in face and scalp lacerations. Am J Emerg Med 13:151–154, 1995.
17. Buckley, MM, and Benfield, P: Eutectic lidocaine/prilocaine cream. A review of the topical anaesthetic/analgesic efficacy of a eutectic mixture of local anaesthetics (EMLA). Drugs 46:126–151, 1993.
18. Zempsky, WT, and Karasic, RB: EMLA versus TAC for topical anesthesia of extremity wounds in children. Ann Emerg Med 30:163–166, 1997.
19. Hardison, CD: Application of a versatile instrument for the production of cutaneous anesthesia without needle penetration of the skin. J Am Coll Emerg Phys 6:266–268, 1977.
20. Greenbaum, SS, and Bernstein, EF: Comparison of iontophoresis of lidocaine with a eutectic mixture of lidocaine and prilocaine (EMLA) for topically administered local anesthesia. J Dermatol Surg Oncol 20:579–583, 1994.
21. Knoop, K, Trott, A, and Syverud, S: Comparison of digital versus metacarpal blocks for repair of finger injuries. Ann Emerg Med 23:1296–1300, 1994.
22. Bartfield, JM, Ford, DT, and Homer, PJ: Buffered versus plain lidocaine for digital nerve blocks. Ann Emerg Med 22:216–219, 1993.
23. Lynch, MT, et al: Comparison of intraoral and percutaneous approaches for infraorbital nerve block. Acad Emerg Med 1:514–519, 1994.
24. Syverud, SA, et al: A comparative study of the percutaneous versus intraoral technique for mental nerve block. Acad Emerg Med 1:509–513, 1994.
25. Scott, DB, et al: Factors affecting plasma levels of lignocaine and prilocaine. Br J Anaesth 44:1040–1049, 1972.
26. Chandler, MJ, Grammer, LC, and Patterson, R: Provocative challenge with local anesthetics in patients with a prior history of reaction. J All Clin Immunol 79:883–886, 1987.
27. Green, SM, Rothrock, SG, and Gorchynski, J: Validation of diphenhydramine as a dermal local anesthetic. Ann Emerg Med 23:1284–1289, 1994.
28. Singer, AJ, and Hollander, JE: Infiltration pain and local anesthetic effects of buffered vs plain 1% diphenhydramine. Acad Emerg Med 2:884–888, 1995.

29. Martin, S, and Wilson, L: Benzyl alcohol with epinephrine as an alternative local anesthetic. Ann Emerg Med 33:495–499, 1999.
30. Bartfield, JM, Weeks Jandreau, S, and Raccio-Roback, N: A randomized trial of diphenhydramine versus benzyl alcohol with epinephrine as an alternative to lidocaine local anesthesia. Ann Emerg Med 32:650–654, 1998.
31. Kimura, ET, et al: Parenteral toxicity studies with benzyl alcohol. Toxicol Appl Pharmacol 18:54–61, 1971.
32. Bartfield, JM, May-Wheeling, HE, Raccio-Robak N, et al: Benzyl alcohol with epinephrine as an alternative local anesthetic to lidocaine with epinephrine. Acad Emerg Med 6:496, 1999.

STEVEN M. GREEN, MD
BARUCH KRAUSS, MD, EDM

CHAPTER

5

Procedural Sedation and Analgesia

Most wounds in older children and adults can be readily repaired without procedural sedation. Skilled practitioners can supplement careful local anesthesia with distraction techniques and a calm, reassuring bedside manner, which are usually sufficient for typical lacerations in older, more cooperative patients. In certain situations, however, patients may require analgesia, anxiolysis, immobilization without sedation, or a combination of these. Specific sedation strategies should be tailored to the unique needs of each patient. Wounds in infants and toddlers often cannot be repaired either technically or humanely without procedural sedation and analgesia (PSA) (Table 5–1).[1,2]

The safety of PSA techniques performed by emergency physicians has been well documented in numerous large series in both children and adults.[1–5] **Successful and safe application of PSA requires careful patient selection, customization of therapy to the specific needs of the patient, and careful patient monitoring for adverse effects.**[2,5,6] PSA should always be performed in accordance with the appropriate specialty guidelines and hospital sedation protocols. Presedation evaluations are required for optimal safety, and the time and nature of the patient's last oral intake should be considered in planning PSA timing and depth. Mandatory elements of monitoring are continuous pulse oximetry and continuous interactive monitoring by a nurse or other health professional capable of rapidly identifying and treating cardiorespiratory complications. PSA requires a minimum of two experienced individuals, most frequently one physician and one nurse.

When anxiolysis alone is the primary objective (with cooperative patients, especially for minor wounds), midazolam by the oral, nasal, rectal, or intravenous (IV) route is the preferred agent, with nitrous oxide as an alternative. For PSA in which analgesia, sedation, immobilization, or a combination of these is required, a combination of midazolam and fentanyl is the most com-

TABLE 5-1. INDICATIONS FOR PROCEDURAL SEDATION AND ANALGESIA IN WOUND REPAIR IN CHILDREN

PSA Frequently Needed

- Complex facial lacerations
- Animal bites of the face requiring extensive irrigation
- Digit lacerations
- Nailbed lacerations
- Wounds in infants and early toddlers
- Chin lacerations (in which repair takes place within the patient's visual field)
- Nasal lacerations
- Periorbital lacerations: Eyelid, eyebrow, and infraorbital rim
- Perioral and oral lacerations: Vermilion border, outer and inner lip, tongue, and corners of the mouth
- Perineal or genital lacerations (straddle injuries)
- Burn débridement
- Highly anxious teenagers and adults
- Uncooperative psychiatric patients
- Mentally challenged patients

PSA Rarely Needed

- Scalp wounds amenable to staples
- Facial wounds amenable to tissue adhesives

monly preferred regimen. IV titration of these agents permits optimal customization of sedation and analgesia to a given patient's needs with a wide safety margin. Ketamine is a safe alternative that more consistently provides the immobilization needed for painful or emotionally disturbing procedures (Fig. 5–1).

INDICATIONS

Situations that require PSA can be divided into three categories:

1. **Insufficient analgesia:** Even in cooperative patients, some wounds are difficult to anesthetize effectively with local agents, so the addition of systemic analgesia is necessary. Examples include larger or deeper wounds, wounds in sensitive areas (e.g., the genitalia or perineum), wounds that require scrubbing (e.g., "road rash"), and burn débridement.
2. **Insufficient anxiolysis:** Some patients are so frightened that procedures cannot be technically or humanely performed without PSA even when the wound is anesthetized. Younger children requiring laceration repair are frequently terrified, and older children and adults may be highly anxious in anticipation of laceration repairs in sensitive or personal regions (e.g., the face, genitalia, perineum).

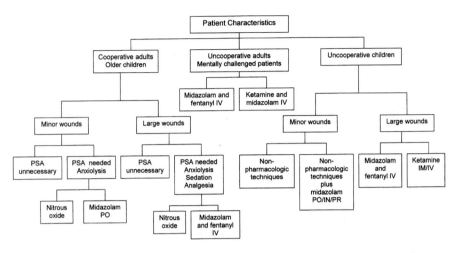

FIG. 5–1. PSA drug selection strategy. PO = oral; PR = rectal; IN = intranasal; IV = intravenous.

3. **Insufficient immobilization:** Repair of complex facial lacerations requires substantial immobilization for optimal cosmesis, and PSA may be indicated solely to prevent excessive motion in such circumstances. Immobilization is most commonly an issue with younger children and mentally challenged individuals.

TECHNIQUE

The depth of sedation is best thought of as a continuum that ranges from mild sedation or analgesia on one end of the spectrum to general anesthesia on the other. This sedation continuum is not drug specific; varying states from mild sedation to general anesthesia can be achieved with all opioids and sedative/hypnotics.

Many practitioners will wish to confine their sedation practice to a primary sedation state, variously known as *procedural sedation, sedation/analgesia,* or *conscious sedation* (Table 5–2). All three terms refer to a depth of sedation at which patients are not reasonably expected to experience cardiorespiratory depression and thus are at minimal risk of complications when appropriate precautions are in place.

Most wound care in cooperative patients can be performed either without sedation or with PSA at a sedation level consistent with these primary states. However, for uncooperative patients such as frightened children, this degree of sedation is commonly insufficient for effective anxiolysis and immobilization, and a deeper level of sedation is required. Deeper sedation of course requires more advanced monitoring, as discussed in the next section.

TABLE 5–2. DEFINITIONS OF SEDATION STATES ACCORDING TO SPECIALTY SOCIETIES

Primary Sedation State (Differing Definitions)

Procedural sedation (American College of Emergency Physicians): "A technique of administering sedatives or dissociative agents with or without analgesics to induce a state that allows the patient to tolerate unpleasant procedures while maintaining cardiorespiratory function. Procedural sedation and analgesia is intended to result in a depressed level of consciousness but one that allows the patient to maintain airway control independently and continuously. Specifically, the drugs, doses, and techniques used are not likely to produce a loss of protective airway reflexes."

Sedation or analgesia (American Society of Anesthesiologists): "A state that allows patients to tolerate unpleasant procedures while maintaining adequate cardiorespiratory function and the ability to respond purposefully to verbal command and/or tactile stimulation. Note that patients whose only response is reflex withdrawal from a painful stimulus are sedated to a greater degree than encompassed by sedation/analgesia."

Conscious sedation (American Academy of Pediatrics): "A medically controlled state of depressed consciousness that (1) allows protective reflexes to be maintained; (2) retains the patient's ability to maintain a patent airway independently and continuously; and (3) permits appropriate response by the patient to physical stimulation or verbal command, e.g., 'open your eyes.'"

Intermediate Sedation State

Deep sedation (American Academy of Pediatrics): "A medically controlled state of depressed consciousness or unconsciousness from which the patient is not easily aroused. It may be accompanied by a partial or complete loss of protective reflexes, and includes the inability to maintain a patent airway independently and respond purposefully to physical stimulation or verbal command."

Anesthetic State

General anesthesia (American Academy of Pediatrics): "A medically controlled state of unconsciousness accompanied by a loss of protective reflexes, including the inability to maintain a patent airway independently and respond purposefully to physical stimulation or verbal command."

Source: Adapted with permission from Krauss, B, and Green, SM: Sedation and analgesia for procedures in children. N Engl J Med 342:939, 2000.

PERSONNEL SKILLS AND TRAINING

The PSA environment must include personnel trained in the rapid identification and treatment of cardiorespiratory complications such as apnea, respiratory depression, partial airway obstruction, emesis, and hypersalivation. These individuals should be proficient at maintaining airway patency and assisting ventilation if needed, and they should be trained in the pharmacology of sedatives and reversal agents. **PSA requires a minimum of two experienced individuals, most frequently one physician and one other health care practitioner, such as a nurse.** The physician oversees drug administration and performs the procedure while the nurse continuously monitors the patient for potential complications and documents medications administered, response to sedation, and periodic vital signs. The nurse must be able to continuously observe the patient's face, mouth, and chest wall motion, so equipment or sterile drapes must not interfere with such visualization. The nurse may assist with minor, interruptible tasks, but the nurse's focus on the patient's cardiopulmonary status must not be impeded. The immediate availability of an individual with advanced life support skills is strongly recommended for primary sedation states, and it is necessary when deeper sedation is likely or possible.

During *deep sedation*, the individual dedicated to patient monitoring should be experienced with this depth of sedation and have no other responsibilities that would interfere with the advanced level of monitoring and documentation appropriate for this sedation level.[7] Sedation policies of individual hospitals may have other requirements for how and when deep sedation is administered based on specific needs and available expertise.

PRESEDATION EVALUATION AND PREPARATION

A directed history and physical examination should precede PSA, including an assessment of underlying medical conditions (Table 5–3), medications, allergies, previous adverse experience with PSA or general anesthesia, time and nature of last oral intake, assessment of heart and lung sounds, and evaluation of the airway for abnormalities that might impair a resuscitation.

The risks, benefits, and limitations of any PSA should be discussed in advance with the patient (or the parent or guardian of a child), and verbal agreement should be obtained. For elective PSA, the American Society of Anesthesiologists recommends an adult fasting guideline of 2 to 3 hours for clear liquids and 6 to 8 hours for solids and nonclear liquids. For children, they recommend an age-stratified fasting guideline of 2 to 3 hours for clear liquids and 4 to 8 hours for solids and nonclear liquids. Nevertheless, the data in the literature are insufficient to test the hypothesis that fasting before a procedure decreases the incidence of adverse outcomes. If the patient does not meet the fasting guidelines, the potential for pulmonary aspiration must be balanced with the timing of the procedure and the required depth of sedation. The risk of wound infection and suboptimal cosmesis increases substantially with delays in repair, and because wound care is accordingly not elective, practitioners need to violate these fasting guidelines almost routinely. A small snack or beverage 1 hour before presentation, for example, should not preclude repair of a small but dirty hand laceration. Delaying irrigation and repair of this wound significantly increases the risk of infection, and the depth of sedation needed should be low enough to entail a minimal risk of impaired airway reflexes. On the other hand, prompt sedation would be unwise for repair of a large scalp laceration in a frightened child if he or she had just eaten a large

TABLE 5–3. PHYSICAL STATUS CLASSIFICATION OF THE AMERICAN SOCIETY OF ANESTHESIOLOGISTS (ASA)

ASA Class	Description	Examples	Suitability for Sedation
1	A normally healthy patient	Unremarkable medical history	Excellent
2	A patient with mild systemic disease; no functional limitation	Mild asthma, controlled seizure disorder, anemia, controlled diabetes mellitus	Generally good
3	A patient with severe systemic disease; definite functional limitation	Moderate to severe asthma, poorly controlled seizure disorder, pneumonia, poorly controlled diabetes mellitus, moderate obesity	Intermediate to poor; consider benefits relative to risks
4	A patient with severe systemic disease that is a constant threat to life	Severe bronchopulmonary dysplasia; sepsis; advanced degrees of pulmonary, cardiac, hepatic, renal, or endocrine insufficiency	Poor; benefits rarely outweigh risks
5	A moribund patient who is not expected to survive without the operation	Septic shock; severe trauma	Extremely poor

Source: Reproduced with permission from Krauss, B, and Green, SM: Sedation and analgesia for procedures in children. N Engl J Med 342:939, 2000.

meal 1 hour before. This wound is at low risk for infection or adverse cosmetic outcome, and a delay of 2 to 4 hours would add a substantially higher margin of safety.

MONITORING

The sedation area should be stocked with age-appropriate equipment for airway management and resuscitation, including a bag-valve mask, oxygen, suction, and intubation supplies. **Continuous pulse oximetry with an audible and visual signal should be routine.** Continuous electrocardiographic (ECG) monitoring is also simple, inexpensive, and readily available. The addition of newer capnographic devices is desirable because end-tidal CO_2 measurements can alert practitioners to respiratory depression and apnea before hypoxemia develops. Vital signs should be periodically measured, including measurements at baseline, after drug administration, on completion of the procedure, during early recovery, and at completion of recovery. **The risk of cardiopulmonary depression is greatest shortly after IV medications are administered and immediately after the procedure, when external stimuli cease.**

When sedation is initiated by the intramuscular (IM), oral, nasal, or rectal routes, it is not mandatory to have IV access. However, an individual skilled in initiating such access should be immediately available.

DISCHARGE

Monitoring after PSA should continue until patients are no longer at risk for cardiorespiratory depression. **To be discharged, patients should be alert and oriented (or returned to age-appropriate baseline), and vital signs should be stable. For children, it should be ensured that a reliable adult will observe each child after discharge for postprocedure complications.**

PROCEDURAL SEDATION AND ANALGESIA DRUGS

As shown in Table 5–4, the current pharmacopoeia of PSA includes the sedative/hypnotic benzodiazepines (midazolam), the analgesic opioids (fentanyl, morphine, meperidine) and their reversal agents (naloxone, flumazenil), a dissociative agent (ketamine), and an inhalational agent (nitrous oxide). Barbiturates and chloral hydrate no longer have a role in PSA for wound care, and their use is now limited to sedation for diagnostic imaging studies.

MIDAZOLAM

Midazolam is the most commonly used PSA agent in both children and adults, and it has an extensive track record of safety. This short-acting benzodiazepine provides potent sedation, amnesia, and anxiolysis and can be administered by multiple routes. **Midazolam is preferred over longer-acting benzodiazepines such as diazepam and lorazepam because of its short duration and versatile routes of administration. The cardiopulmonary depressant effects of midazolam can be reversed with the antagonist flumazenil.**[8,9]

Midazolam can be readily administered by the oral, nasal, or rectal route for minor wounds in which anxiolysis is the primary objective.[10,11] Benzodiazepines provide no analgesia, however, and for larger wounds or those in which more reliable and potent sedation is necessary, an IV should be placed and midazolam should be titrated to effect. An opioid (most commonly fentanyl) can thus be readily coadministered to achieve balanced sedation and analgesia.

The synergistic respiratory depressant effect of concurrent benzodiazepines and opioids must be respected, and doses and speed of titration adjusted downward accordingly.[12]

FENTANYL

For wound care, the short-acting opioid fentanyl is preferred to the long-acting meperidine and morphine, owing to its faster onset, shorter duration, and lack of histamine release. Fentanyl has an extensive track record of safety when carefully titrated by the IV route, and co-administration with midazolam permits optimal customization of sedation and analgesia to a given patient's needs. Fentanyl delivery by the oral transmucosal route (i.e., lozenges) initially appeared promising, but unacceptably high rates of emesis (31 percent to 45 percent) have limited the popularity of this technique.[13,14]

Morphine and meperidine remain the preferred agents for analgesia of longer duration. The cardiopulmonary depressant effects of opioids can be reversed with the antagonist naloxone.[15]

KETAMINE

When administered through the IM or IV route, ketamine rapidly produces a trance-like cataleptic condition characterized by profound analgesia, sedation, amnesia, and immobilization. This unique "dissociative state" permits painful procedures to be performed more consistently and effectively than with other PSA agents but does not compromise upper airway muscular tone and protective airway reflexes. Normal spontaneous respirations are essentially always maintained, but rapid IV administration can cause transient respiratory depression and apnea. Therefore, slow IV administration is recommended.

Unpleasant hallucinations and dreams during the recovery period have substantially limited the use of ketamine in adults, but such emergence reactions are quite rare in children and are far milder when they do occur.[4,16–18] Concurrent benzodiazepine treatment has been shown to minimize unpleasant hallucinatory reactions in adults, but this intervention shows no apparent benefit in children.[18] Clinicians can readily treat such reactions with midazolam on the rare occasions when they do occur in children.

For many physicians, ketamine is the preferred agent for facilitating treatment of larger wounds in children when substantial analgesia and reliable immobilization are necessary. Because of the profound analgesia characteristic of the dissociative state, local anesthesia is usually unnecessary. Clinicians administering ketamine must be especially knowledgeable about the unique actions and numerous contraindications of this drug (see Table 5–4).

The safety of ketamine has been extensively documented. Owing to its safety, efficacy, and simplicity of administration, ketamine enjoys wide ongoing use throughout the developing world and in veterinary medicine. Ketamine may be preferred over other PSA agents when fasting is not assured because protective airway reflexes are preserved when it is used. In almost 30 years of regular use, there are no reports of clinically significant ketamine-associated aspiration in patients lacking established contraindications.

TABLE 5–4. PROCEDURAL SEDATION AND ANALGESIA DRUG DOSING RECOMMENDATIONS FOR WOUND REPAIR[a]

Drug	Clinical Effects	Adult Dose[b]	Pediatric Dose	Onset, min	Duration, min	Comments
Sedative/Hypnotics						
Midazolam[c] (Versed)	Sedation, motion control, anxiolysis No analgesia Reversible with flumazenil	IV: Initial 1 mg, then titrated to max 5 mg IM: 5 mg or 0.07 mg/kg IM	IV (0.5–5.0 years): Initial 0.05–0.10 mg/kg, then titrated to max 0.6 mg/kg IV (6–12 year): Initial 0.025–0.050 mg/kg, then titrated to max 0.4 mg/kg IM: 0.10–0.15 mg/kg; PO: 0.50–0.75 mg/kg IN: 0.2–0.5 mg/kg; PR: 0.25–0.50 mg/kg	IV: 2–3 IM: 10–20 PO: 15–30 IN: 10–15 PR: 10–30	IV: 45–60 IM: 60–120 PO: 60–90 IN: 60 PR: 60–90	Reduce dose when used in combination with opioids. May produce paradoxical excitement. Because drugs cannot be titrated with the oral, rectal, or intranasal routes, monitor closely for oversedation.
Analgesic[d]						
Fentanyl (Sublimaze)	Analgesia Reversible with naloxone	IV: 50 mcg, may repeat q3min, titrate to effect	IV: 1.0 mcg/kg/dose, may repeat q3 min, titrate to effect	IV: 3–5	IV: 30–60	Reduce dosing when combined with midazolam.
Dissociative Agent						
Ketamine (Ketalar)	Analgesia, dissociation, amnesia, motion control	Limited experience in ED setting	IV: 1.0–1.5 mg/kg slowly over 1–2 min, may repeat half dose q10min prn IM: 4–5 mg/kg; may repeat after 10 min	IV: 1 IM: 3–5	IV: dissociation 15; recovery 60 IM: dissociation 15–30; recovery 90–150	Multiple contraindications.[e] Risk of unpleasant hallucinations or dreams if age older than 15 years (rare if younger), which may be blunted with use of midazolam. Hypersalivation can be minimized with concurrent atropine 0.01 mg/kg IM/IV (min 0.1 mg; max 0.5 mg).

Source: Adapted with permission from Krauss, B, and Green, SM: Sedation and analgesia for procedures in children. N Engl J Med 342:942–942, 2000. Copyright © 2000 Massachusetts Medical Society. All rights reserved.

Inhalational Agent

Nitrous oxide (Nitronox)	Anxiolysis, analgesia, sedation, amnesia (all mild)	Preset mixture with minimum 40% O₂ self-administered by demand valve mask (requires cooperative patient)		< 5	< 5 after discontinuation	Requires specialized apparatus and gas scavenger capability. Several contraindications.[f] Synergistic effect with recent opioids or sedative/hypnotics; use with caution in this setting.

Reversal Agents (Antagonists)

Naloxone (Narcan)	Opioid reversal	IV/IM: 0.4–2.0 mg	IV/IM: 0.1 mg/kg/dose up to max of 2 mg/dose; may repeat q2 min prn	IV: 2	IV: 20–40 IM: 60–90	If shorter acting than the reversed drug, serial doses may be required.
Flumazenil (Romazicon)	Benzodiazepine reversal	IV: 0.2 mg; may repeat q1min up to 1 mg	IV: 0.02 mg/kg/dose; may repeat q1 min up to 1 mg	IV: 1–2	IV: 30–60	If shorter acting than the reversed drug, serial doses may be required. Do not use in patients receiving chronic benzodiazepines, cyclosporine, isoniazid, lithium, propoxyphene, theophylline, TCAs.

[a] Alterations in dosing may be indicated based on the clinical situation and the practitioner's experience with these agents. Individual dosages may vary when used in combination with other agents, especially when benzodiazepines are combined with opioids.

[b] Use lower doses in geriatric patients and those with significant cardiopulmonary disease.

[c] Midazolam is preferred to other benzodiazepines (e.g., diazepam, lorazepam) for PSA because of its shorter duration of action and multiple routes of administration.

[d] Fentanyl is preferred to other opioids (e.g., morphine, meperidine) for PSA because of its faster onset, shorter recovery time, and lack of histamine release.

[e] Generally accepted contraindications to ketamine: Age < 3 months; history of airway instability, tracheal surgery, or tracheal stenosis; procedures involving stimulation of the posterior pharynx; active pulmonary infection or disease (including active upper respiratory infection); cardiovascular disease (including angina, heart failure, or hypertension); significant head injury, central nervous system masses, or hydrocephalus; glaucoma or acute globe injury; psychosis; porphyria; thyroid disorder or thyroid medication.

[f] Generally accepted contraindications to nitrous oxide: Pregnancy (patient or personnel); preexisting nausea or vomiting; trapped gas pockets (e.g., middle ear infection, pneumothorax, bowel obstruction).

IV = intravenous; IM = intramuscular; IN = intranasal; PO = oral; PR = rectal; TCA = tricyclic antidepressant.

An antisialogogue (e.g., atropine, glycopyrrolate) is typically co-administered with ketamine to minimize the hypersalivation occasionally observed with this drug. Whether such prophylaxis is routinely necessary remains unclear and unstudied, but most authors recommend regular co-administration of antisialogogues, which are safe, simple, and widely used for this purpose.

NITROUS OXIDE

Nitrous oxide gas is easy to use, non-invasive, and provides rapid onset and recovery. It is blended with oxygen using a flowmeter, or dispensed in a preset mixture with a minimum of 40 percent oxygen. Self-administration by demand valve mask has been shown to be extremely safe, but the degree of cooperation required limits its use to adults and older children. Self-administration also provides a built-in fail-safe mechanism because oversedation causes the patient to drop the mask and terminate gas delivery. Because of the necessity of using a mask, facial lacerations cannot be readily repaired with this technique. In the concentrations used with self-administration, nitrous oxide is a weak analgesic and sedative; therefore, it is most useful as an anxiolytic.[19–21]

REVERSAL AGENTS (ANTAGONISTS)

The availability of specific opioid and benzodiazepine antagonists permits oversedation and respiratory depression to be rapidly reversed when needed during PSA (see Table 5–4).[22–25]

SELECTION STRATEGIES FOR PROCEDURAL SEDATION AND ANALGESIA DRUGS

Clinicians must customize their PSA drug selection based on the unique needs of the patient (i.e., anxiolysis, analgesia, immobilization) and their individual level of experience with specific agents (see Fig. 5–1).

MINOR WOUNDS IN COOPERATIVE ADULTS AND OLDER CHILDREN

Sedation is typically unnecessary in these situations. Mild anxiolysis with nitrous oxide or midazolam can frequently make patients more comfortable.

LARGE WOUNDS IN COOPERATIVE ADULTS AND OLDER CHILDREN

Supplementation of local anesthesia with midazolam and fentanyl titrated IV permits ready customization of sedation depth and pain relief to the specific needs of each patient. Nitrous oxide alone is sufficient in many cases.

WOUNDS IN UNCOOPERATIVE ADULTS AND MENTALLY CHALLENGED INDIVIDUALS

Regardless of their size, wounds in uncooperative adult-sized patients are difficult to repair without sedation. Depending on operator experience, midazolam/fentanyl or ketamine may be used in these situations. Midazolam and fentanyl can be titrated IV to a relatively deep level of sedation, but it must be recognized that the risk of adverse effects increases with sedation depth. Ketamine can also provide the profound analgesia and immobilization necessary to perform extremely painful procedures, but it does present the risk of unpleasant hallucinatory recovery reactions, as previously discussed. These reactions can be blunted with the use of a benzodiazepine (most commonly midazolam). **Ketamine should be used only with extreme caution in older adults because its sympathomimetic properties may aggravate underlying coronary artery disease or hypertension.** Occasionally, large wounds in uncooperative adults are better managed in the operating room with general anesthesia.

MINOR WOUNDS IN UNCOOPERATIVE CHILDREN

Skilled practitioners often can manage trivial lacerations in uncooperative children by using a combination of distraction techniques; comforting; careful local anesthesia; and, when necessary, brief, forcible immobilization. In other cases, supplementing nonpharmacologic techniques with midazolam anxiolysis may be sufficient to permit successful wound repair. Although oral administration is most popular, the nasal or rectal routes can also be used, depending on operator experience and preference.

LARGE WOUNDS IN UNCOOPERATIVE CHILDREN

In many centers, ketamine is regarded as the best option in such children because the dissociative state can consistently provide the immobilization and analgesia needed for such repairs. Practitioners inexperienced with ketamine may use midazolam and fentanyl titrated to deep levels of sedation to perform such procedures.

INCISION AND DRAINAGE OF ABSCESSES

Abscess incision and drainage, especially the drainage and packing of the wound, can be extremely painful. Therefore, it requires both pain control and a reasonable degree of immobilization for success and patient comfort. Smaller abscesses in cooperative patients can sometimes be drained using local anesthesia alone, but most abscesses require either IV midazolam and fentanyl or nitrous oxide in adults or ketamine in children and mentally challenged individuals.

FOREIGN BODY REMOVAL

Many subcutaneous foreign bodies can be removed from cooperative patients using local anesthesia alone. Because immobilization is frequently critical to procedural success, uncooperative subjects may require ketamine or titration of midazolam and fentanyl to a substantial depth of sedation.

BURN DÉBRIDEMENT

Débridement of more than minimal burns is exquisitely painful, so patients undergoing the procedure require significant analgesia either with ketamine or with fentanyl and midazolam. Nitrous oxide in concentrations attainable with hand-held mask delivery is unlikely to provide sufficient analgesia.

REFERENCES

1. Krauss, B, and Green, SM: Procedural sedation and analgesia in children. N Engl J Med 342:938–945, 2000.
2. American College of Emergency Physicians: Clinical policy for procedural sedation and analgesia in the emergency department. Ann Emerg Med 31:663–677, 1998.
3. Pena, BMG, and Krauss, B: Complications of procedural sedation and analgesia in a pediatric emergency department. Ann Emerg Med 34:483–490, 1999.
4. Green, SM, Rothrock, SG, Lynch, EL, et al: Intramuscular ketamine for pediatric sedation in the emergency department: Safety profile with 1,022 cases. Ann Emerg Med 31:688–697, 1998.
5. American Society of Anesthesiologists: Practice guidelines for sedation and analgesia by non-anesthesiologists. Anesthesiology 84:459–471, 1996.
6. American Academy of Pediatrics Committee on Drugs: Guidelines for monitoring and management of pediatric patients during and after sedation for diagnostic and therapeutic procedures. Pediatrics 89:1110–1115, 1992.
7. Krauss, B, Shannon, MW, Damian, FJ, et al: Guidelines for Pediatric Sedation, ed 2. American College of Emergency Physicians, Dallas, Tex, 1998.
8. Sievers, TD, Yee, JD, Foley, ME, et al: Midazolam for conscious sedation during pediatric oncology procedures: Safety and recovery parameters. Pediatrics 88:1172–1179, 1991.
9. Reves, JG, Fragen, RJ, Vinik, HR, et al: Midazolam: Pharmacology and uses. Anesthesiology 63:310–324, 1985.
10. Connors, K, and Terndrup, TE: Nasal versus oral midazolam for sedation of anxious children undergoing laceration repair. Ann Emerg Med 24:1074–1079, 1994.
11. Theroux, MC, West, DW, Corddry, DH, et al: Efficacy of intranasal midazolam in facilitating the suturing of lacerations in preschool children in the emergency room. Pediatrics 91:624–627, 1993.
12. Bailey, PL, Pace, NL, Ashburn, MA, et al. Frequent hypoxemia and apnea after sedation with midazolam and fentanyl. Anesthesiology 73:826–830, 1990.
13. Green, SM, Rothrock, SG, Harris, T, et al: Intravenous ketamine for pediatric sedation in the emergency department: safety and efficacy with 156 cases. Acad Emerg Med 5:971–976, 1998.
14. Dachs, RJ, and Innes, GM: Intravenous ketamine sedation of pediatric patients in the emergency department. Ann Emerg Med 29:146–150, 1997.
15. Epstein, RH, Mendel, HG, Witkowski, TA, et al: The safety and efficacy of oral transmucosal fentanyl citrate for preoperative sedation in young children. Anesth Analg 83:1200–1205, 1996.
16. Green, SM, and Johnson, NE: Ketamine sedation for pediatric procedures: Part 2, Review and implications. Ann Emerg Med 19:1033–1046, 1990.
17. Green, SM, Nakamura, R, and Johnson, NE: Ketamine sedation for pediatric procedures: Part 1, A prospective series. Ann Emerg Med 19:1024–1032, 1990.
18. Sherwin, TS, Green, SM, Khan A, et al: Does adjunctive midazolam reduce recovery agitation

after ketamine sedation for pediatric procedures? A randomized, double-blind, placebo-controlled trial. Ann Emerg Med 35:229–238, 2000.

19. Gamis, AS, Knapp, JF, and Glenski, JA: Nitrous oxide analgesia in a pediatric emergency department. Ann Emerg Med 18:177–181, 1989.
20. Burton, JH, Auble, TE, and Fuchs, SM: Effectiveness of 50% nitrous oxide/50% oxygen during laceration repair in children. Acad Emerg Med 5:112–117, 1998.
21. Luhmann, JD, Kennedy, RM, Porter, FL, et al: A randomized clinical trial of continuous-flow nitrous oxide and midazolam for sedation of young children during laceration repair. Ann Emerg Med 37:20–27, 2001.
22. Chudnofsky, CR, for the Emergency Medicine Conscious Sedation Study Group: Safety and efficacy of flumazenil in reversing conscious sedation in the emergency department. Acad Emerg Med 4:944–950, 1997.
23. Handal, KA, Schauban, JL, and Salamone, FR: Naloxone. Ann Emerg Med 12:438–445, 1983.
24. Longnecker, DE, Grazis, PA, and Eggers, GWN: Naloxone for antagonism of morphine-induced respiratory depression. Anesth Analg (Cleve) 52:447–453, 1973.
25. Shannon, M, Albers, G, Burkhart, K, et al: Safety and efficacy of flumazenil in the reversal of benzodiazepine-induced conscious sedation. J Pediatr 131:582–586, 1997.

JUDD E. HOLLANDER, MD

C H A P T E R

6

Wound Closure Options

Most lacerations heal without sequelae, but mismanagement may lead to wound infections, prolonged convalescence, and unsightly and dysfunctional scars. **The goals of wound management are simple: avoid infection and achieve a functional and aesthetically pleasing scar.**[1] These goals may be accomplished by reducing tissue contamination, débriding devitalized tissue, restoring perfusion in poorly perfused wounds, and achieving a well-approximated tension-free skin closure.

The advantages and disadvantages of the currently available wound closure methods are presented in Table 6–1. Preferred methods of wound closure based on the type of wound are presented in Table 6–2. This chapter presents a general overview of the various wound closure methods, which are discussed in more detail in subsequent chapters.

TIMING OF WOUND CLOSURE

Most lacerations require primary closure. Primary closure results in more rapid healing and less patient discomfort than secondary closure. The time interval from injury to closure of a laceration is directly related to the risk of subsequent infection, but the length of this "golden period" is highly variable.[5-7] In one study of 300 hand and forearm lacerations, Morgan and colleagues[5] found that lacerations closed within 4 hours had a 7 percent infection rate compared with a 21 percent infection rate for those closed more than 4 hours after injury. On the other hand, in a study of 2834 pediatric patients, Baker and Lanuti[6] found that the infection rate for lacerations closed more than 6 hours after the time of injury was no greater than the rate for lacerations closed within 6 hours. The most widely quoted study[7] comes from Jamaica, where the authors used healing (defined as epithelialization without infection) as the main outcome. This study of 204 lacerations found that facial lacerations healed well regardless of the time to closure. In contrast, lacerations of the trunk or ex-

Humans have managed wounds from the beginning of civilization. The first evidence of wounds can be found in our ancestor, *Australopithecus africans*, who was present over 5 million years ago.[2] The first written records of wounds date back to 2500 BC.[3] Initial treatments for wounds consisted of herbal balms or draughts with application of leaves or grasses as bandages. Ointments were made from a wide variety of animal, vegetable, and mineral substances. Wounds were mostly left open, but wound closure using the jaws of ants was used by some cultures (see Chapter 8).[4] The world's oldest suture was placed by an embalmer on the abdomen of a mummy in approximately 1100 BC.[2] During early civilization, the care of wounds was dominated by magic and rituals. Celsus first described primary and secondary wound closure more than 2000 years ago.

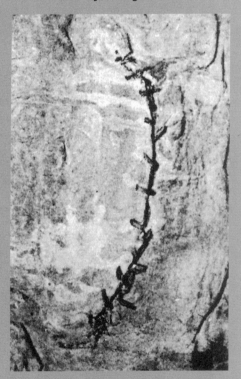

During the Middle Ages, pus was believed to be necessary for healing. As a result, various agents were used to promote suppuration. Advances in the fields of anesthesiology and surgery during the past two centuries and the development of academic emergency medicine in the past decade have led to the development of many of the practices still prevalent today. These practices are based on thorough débridement and cleansing of wounds and the use of aseptic wound closure techniques.

TABLE 6–1. ADVANTAGES AND DISADVANTAGES OF COMMON WOUND CLOSURE TECHNIQUES

Technique	Advantages	Disadvantages
Suture	Time-honored procedure Meticulous closure Greatest tensile strength Lowest dehiscence rate	Requires removal Requires anesthesia Greatest tissue reactivity Highest cost Slowest application
Staples	Rapid application Low tissue reactivity Low cost Low risk of needle-stick injuries	Less meticulous closure May interfere with some older-generation imaging techniques (e.g., CT, MRI)
Tissue adhesives	Rapid application Patient comfort Resistant to bacterial growth No need for removal Low cost No risk of needle-stick injuries	Lower tensile strength than sutures Dehiscence over high-tension areas (e.g., joints) Not useful on hands Patient cannot bathe or swim
Surgical tapes	Least reactive Lowest infection rates Rapid application Patient comfort Low cost No risk of needle-stick	Frequently fall off Lower tensile strength than sutures Highest rate of dehiscence Require use of toxic adjuncts Cannot be used in areas of hair Cannot get wet

Source: Adapted with permission from Hollander, JE, and Singer, AJ: Laceration management. Ann Emerg Med 34:364, 1999.

CT = computed tomography; MRI = magnetic resonance imaging.

tremity had lower rates of healing if they were closed more than 19 hours from the time of injury (63% to 75%) than if they were closed earlier (75% to 91%). The subgroups were small, however, ranging from 8 to 44 patients.[7]

Based on these studies, it seems most prudent to separately consider each individual laceration. **Before closing a wound, consider the time from injury until presentation, etiology, location, degree of contamination, host risk factors, and the importance of cosmetic appearance.** Then it is possible to decide whether or not to perform primary wound closure. For example, a 20-hour-old laceration on the face of a healthy 4-year-old child, which has a low likelihood of infection, may be closed primarily. However, a deep laceration in the foot of a diabetic patient is at increased risk of infection and should not be closed primarily. Thus, the timing during which wound closure is safe needs to be individualized.[1] Wounds that are not closed primarily because of

TABLE 6–2. SELECTION OF WOUND CLOSURE METHOD

Type of Wound	Preferred Closure Method	Alternative Closure Method
Scalp laceration	Staples	Sutures (particularly with deep, bloody wounds)
Non-gaping, superficial facial laceration	Tissue adhesives	Sutures
Gaping or complex facial laceration	Sutures	—
High-tension lacerations	Sutures	Tissue adhesives with immobilization
Hand and foot lacerations	Sutures	—
Avulsion lacerations with fragile skin or tenuous blood supply	Tissue adhesives	Surgical tapes
Long, linear lacerations	Staples	Tissue adhesives

a high risk of infection should be considered for delayed primary closure after 4 days. After 4 days of open wound management, the risk of infection substantially decreases.

METHODS OF WOUND CLOSURE

The ideal wound closure technique would allow a meticulous wound closure, would be easy and rapid to apply, would be painless, would have a low infection rate, would cause no risk to the health care provider, would be inexpensive, and would result in minimal scarring. Sutures are the most commonly used wound closure technique.[8] Tissue adhesives have recently become approved by the Food and Drug Administration and are expected to replace sutures in 25 to 33 percent of emergency department laceration repairs and many surgical incisions.[9] Other alternatives include using staples and surgical tapes.

SUTURES

Sutures are the time-honored and most reliable method of wound closure. They produce a meticulous wound closure with the greatest tensile strength and the lowest likelihood of dehiscence. Even the most complex laceration can be well approximated by suturing. Nonabsorbable sutures retain most of their tensile strength for more than 60 days, are relatively nonreactive, and are appropriate for closure of the outermost layer of the laceration or for repair of tendons.[10–12] However, the need for removal of nonabsorbable sutures is a disadvantage.

Absorbable sutures are usually used to close structures that are deeper than the epidermis. Most absorbable sutures increase up to 1 month the duration of time that the wound retains 50 percent of its tensile strength. Some synthetic absorbable sutures retain their tensile strength for as long as 2 months, making them useful in areas with high-dynamic and static tensions.

Deep sutures can be used to relieve skin tension and should be used to decrease dead space and hematoma formation. They may improve cosmetic outcome. Many advise the use of deep sutures to reduce scar width (especially on the face), but little evidence supports this recommendation. In fact, a study comparing closure of laminectomy incisions with and without deep sutures failed to demonstrate any differences in scar width.[13] Animal studies[14,15] suggest that deep sutures should be avoided in highly contaminated wounds, where they increase the risk of infection. Although the use of absorbable sutures is generally reserved for the subcuticular tissues, rapidly dissolving forms can be used to close the skin of children in order to avoid the discomfort associated with suture removal.[16,17]

Suture closure does have several disadvantages. Local anesthesia is needed to decrease the pain of the suturing. Suture placement is also the most time-consuming wound closure option. Sutures produce more tissue reactivity and inflammation than any of the other options. The placement of sutures poses a small but real risk of blood and body fluid exposure through skin puncture of the health care provider. If not removed in a timely manner, sutures leave unsightly hatch marks on either side of the wound. The cost and inconvenience of suturing and suture removal may make other wound closure options more attractive for some lacerations and incisions.

STAPLES

Staples are the most rapid method of closure, and they are especially well suited for scalp wounds.[18,19] They are associated with lower rates of foreign body reaction and infection.[18,20,21] Staples also reduce the risk of needle-stick injuries to the health care provider. Brickman and Lambert[21] used staples in 75 patients with 87 lacerations to the scalp, trunk, and extremities. None of the patients developed infections, and only one patient had a dehiscence. Ritchie and Rocke[18] performed a randomized, controlled trial comparing sutures with staples for scalp lacerations. They found that lacerations healed equally well, with low infection rates ($< 2\%$) in both groups. In general, staples are considered particularly useful for scalp,[18,22] trunk, and extremity wounds,[1] and when saving time is essential, such as in mass casualties and in victims of multiple trauma.[1] However, they do not allow as meticulous a closure as sutures, and they are slightly more painful to remove.[19] In animal models, staples are associated with lower rates of bacterial growth and lower infection rates than sutures.[20] In clinical series,[22] these differences may be statistically significant but have limited clinical significance.

Staple removal requires a special device. These devices are readily available in emergency rooms but are not stocked in all primary care offices. The implications of this situation for postoperative wound care is further discussed in Chapter 17.

ADHESIVE TAPES

Adhesive tapes are associated with the lowest rate of infection, but they tend to slough off with any tension. Advantages of adhesive tapes to the patient and health care provider include rapid application, little or no patient discomfort, low cost, and no risk of needle-stick injuries. They are associated with minimal tissue reactivity and yield the lowest infection rates of any wound closure method. They may be left on for long periods without resulting in suture hatch marks.

Surgical tapes are even less reactive than staples,[20] but they require the use of adhesive adjuncts (e.g., tincture of benzoin), which increases local induration and wound infection.[23] Adhesive adjuncts are toxic to wounds, so care should be taken so they do not enter the wound. Adhesive tapes have the lowest tensile strength of wound closure devices and do not maintain the integrity of wound closure in areas that are subject to tension.[24]

Surgical tapes are seldom recommended for primary wound closure in the emergency department,[1] but they are often used after suture removal to decrease tension on the wound until they fall off. The reasons for very low use rates are high rates of dislodgement and dehiscence, the inability to use them in hair-bearing areas, and the need to keep them dry. Their use is typically reserved for linear lacerations under minimal tension.

Postoperative care of wounds closed with adhesive tapes requires limited movement of the area. The area also should be kept as dry as possible because the presence of moisture may result in rapid tape dislodgement and subsequent wound dehiscence.

TISSUE ADHESIVES

Tissue adhesives provide cost-effective, needle-free, rapid closure of easily approximated wound edges, with long-term cosmesis comparable to 5-0 and 6-0 sutures. Tissue adhesives can be used for lacerations and incisions that have easily apposed wound edges. They may produce a mild burning sensation, but they generally cause less pain than sutures or staples. Medical grade cyanoacrylate adhesives also provide some resistance to bacterial growth.[25] The reduced need for local anesthesia before wound closure and for return visits for removal makes them a more cost-effective wound closure device than sutures or staples.[26] The risk of needle-stick injury to the health care provider is also reduced.

Observational studies of children with small scalp, face, or limb lacerations treated with a butyl-2-cyanoacrylate (Histoacryl Blue; B. Braun, Melsungen, Germany) found low infection rates (< 2%) and dehiscence rates (0.6% to 1.8%). Histoacryl Blue results in similar long-term cosmetic outcomes as 5-0 or 6-0 sutures when used for repair of small facial lacerations.[27] Several clinical studies[28–31] have compared the use of 2-octylcyanoacrylate to 5-0 and 6-0 sutures. In all studies, the 3-month cosmetic outcomes, short-term infection rates, and wound dehiscence rates were all similar when the use of 2-octyl-cyanoacrylate was compared with skin closure with sutures. The time required to close the wound was more than 50 percent shorter in the group treated with

2-octylcyanoacrylate. A recent study[32] found that the use of octylcyanoacrylate adhesives for skin closure after elective facial plastic surgical procedures produced better long-term results than did the use of sutures.

Tissue adhesives are a needle-free alternative to sutures and staples for the closure of many lacerations and surgical incisions. They produce an excellent cosmetic appearance that is comparable to the outcome with sutures. 2-Octylcyanoacrylates can be used in locations that would otherwise be closed with 5-0 or 6-0 nonabsorbable sutures. These adhesives can be used in areas of higher tension only if subcutaneous or subcuticular absorbable sutures are placed to relieve tension on the skin.

The butylcyanoacrylates have less tensile strength than 5-0 sutures and only approximately one third the tensile strength of the octylcyanoacrylates.[1] Their use is restricted to very small facial lacerations.

Tissue adhesives have some disadvantages and limitations. They cannot be used in complex lacerations that cannot be manually approximated. They are not as strong as larger (4-0) sutures. 2-Octylcyanoacrylate adhesives can be used in areas of higher tension only if subcutaneous or subcuticular absorbable sutures are also used to relieve tension on the skin edges. They should not be used over areas subject to great tension or repetitive movement, such as over the joints or hands.[33] Increasing rates and amounts of polymerization may be associated with increased heat sensation by the patient. For optimal results, they should be applied to a bloodless field. If oozing of blood continues, sutures or staples might provide a better alternative.

Butylcyanoacrylate adhesives should not get wet. Patients may shower and wash when using octylcyanoacrylate adhesives, but lacerations should not receive prolonged exposure to water, such as in swimming. When tissue adhesives are used for laceration closure, topical ointments should not be applied. Ointments may loosen the tissue adhesives and may result in dehiscence.

REFERENCES

1. Singer, AJ, Hollander, JE, and Quinn, JV: Evaluation and management of traumatic lacerations. N Engl J Med 337:1142–1148, 1997.
2. Majno, G: The Healing Hand. Man and Wound in the Ancient World. Harvard University Press, Cambridge, Massachusetts, 1975.
3. Forrest, RD: Early history of wound treatment. J Royal Soc Med 75:198–205, 1982.
4. Wheeler, WM: Ants: Their Structure and Behavior. Columbia University Press, New York, 1960.
5. Morgan, WJ, Hutchison, D, and Johnson, HM: The delayed treatment of wounds of the hand and forearm under antibiotic cover. Br J Surg 67:140–141, 1980.
6. Baker, MD, and Lanuti, M: The management and outcome of lacerations in urban children. Ann Emerg Med 19:1001–1005, 1990.
7. Berk, WA, Osbourne, DD, and Taylor, DD: Evaluation of the "golden period" for wound repair: 204 cases from a third-world emergency department. Ann Emerg Med 17:496–500, 1988.
8. Hollander, JE, Singer, AJ, Valentine, S, et al: Wound registry: Development and validation. Ann Emerg Med 25:675–685, 1995.
9. Singer, AJ, and Hollander, JE: Tissue adhesives for laceration closure (letter). JAMA 278:703, 1997.
10. Markovchick, V: Suture materials and mechanical after care. Emerg Med Clin North Am 10:673–688, 1992.
11. Swanson, NA, and Tromovitch, TA: Suture materials, 1980s: Properties, uses, and abuses. Inter J Derm 21:373–378, 1982.

12. Ratner, D, Nelson, BR, and Johnson, TM: Basic suture materials and suturing techniques. Semin Dermatol 13:20–26, 1994.
13. Winn, HR, Jane, JA, Rodeheaver, G, et al: Influence of subcuticular sutures on scar formation. Am J Surg 133:257–259, 1977.
14. Mehta, PH, Dunn, KA, Bradfield, JF, et al: Contaminated wounds: infection rates with subcutaneous sutures. Ann Emerg Med 27:43–48, 1996.
15. deHoll, D, Rodeheaver, G, Edgerton, MT, et al: Potentiation of infection by suture closure of dead space. Am J Surg 127:716–720, 1974.
16. Start, NJ, Armstrong, AM, and Robson, WJ: The use of chromic catgut in the primary closure of scalp wounds in children. Arch Emerg Med 6:216–219, 1989.
17. Tandon, SC, Kelly, J, Turtle, M, et al: Irradiated polyglactin 910: A new synthetic absorbable suture. J R Coll Surg Edinb 40:185–187, 1995.
18. Ritchie, AJ, and Rocke, LG: Staples versus sutures in the closure of scalp wounds: A prospective, double-blind, randomized trial. Injury 20:217–218, 1989.
19. George, TK, and Simpson, DC: Skin wound closure with staples in the accident and emergency department. J Roy Coll Surg Edinburgh 30:54–56, 1985.
20. Johnson, A, Rodeheaver, GT, Durand, LS, et al: Automatic disposable stapling devices for wound closure. Ann Emerg Med 10:631–635, 1981.
21. Brickman, KR, and Lambert, RW. Evaluation of skin stapling for wound closure in the emergency department. Ann Emerg Med 18:1122–1125, 1989.
22. Hollander, JE, Giarrusso, E, Cassara, G, et al: Comparison of staples and sutures for closure of scalp lacerations (abstract). Acad Emerg Med 4:460–461, 1997.
23. Panek, PH, Prusak, MP, Bolt, D, et al: Potentiation of wound infection by adhesive adjuncts. Am Surgeon. June:343–345, 1972.
24. Rothnie, NG, and Taylor, GW: Sutureless skin closure. A clinical trial. Br Med J 2:1027–1030, 1963.
25. Quinn, JV, Ramotar, K, and Osmond, MH: Antimicrobial effects of a new tissue adhesive. Acad Emerg Med 3:536–537, 1996.
26. Osmond, MH, Klassen, TP, and Quinn, JV: Economic comparison of a tissue adhesive and suturing in the repair of pediatric facial lacerations. J Pediatr 126:892–895, 1995.
27. Quinn, JV, Drzewiecki, A, Li, MM, et al: A randomized, controlled trial comparing a tissue adhesive with suturing in the repair of pediatric facial lacerations. Ann Emerg Med 22:1130–1135, 1993.
28. Quinn, JV, Wells, GA, Sutcliffe, T, et al: A randomized trial comparing octylcyanoacrylate tissue adhesive and sutures in the management of traumatic lacerations. JAMA 277:1527–1530, 1997.
29. Quinn, JV, Wells, GA, Sutcliffe, T, et al: Tissue adhesive vs. suture wound repair at one year: randomized clinical trial correlating early, three-month, and one year cosmetic outcome. Ann Emerg Med 32:645–649, 1998.
30. Singer, AJ, Hollander, JE, Valentine, SM, et al: Prospective randomized controlled trial of tissue adhesive (2-octylcyanoacrylate) vs standard wound closure techniques for laceration repair. Acad Emerg Med 5:94–99, 1998.
31. Bruns, TB, Robinson, BS, Smith, RJ, et al: A new tissue adhesive for laceration repair in children. J Pediatr 132:1067–1070, 1998.
32. Toriumi, DM, Ogrady, K, Desai, D, et al: Use of 2-octylcyanoacrylate for skin closure in facial plastic surgery. Plast Reconstr Surg 102:2209–2219, 1998.
33. Saxena, AK, and Willital, GH: Octylcyanoacrylate tissue adhesive in the repair of pediatric extremity lacerations. Am Surg 65:470–472, 1999.

ADAM J. SINGER, MD

CHAPTER

7

Adhesive Tapes

INDICATIONS

The advantages of adhesive tapes include their resistance to infection, ease of application, elimination of suture marks, painless application and removal, and even distribution of tension across the wound (Table 7–1). They are also particularly well suited for closing partially avulsed skin or flap lacerations that may be torn or strangulated with standard sutures. However, because of their tendency to slough off, they should not be used for wounds subject to high tension, over hair-bearing or oily areas, or in uncooperative patients. The indications and contraindications for use of adhesive tapes are presented in Table 7–2.

COMPARISON TO SUTURES

As early as 1933, DuMotier[3] noted that silk-sutured wounds in guinea pigs were susceptible to wound infection. This finding has been confirmed in later studies,[4–6] which have demonstrated that the incidence of infection of contaminated wounds closed with adhesive tape is considerably less than the incidence for such wounds closed with sutures. Analysis of healing surgical incisions closed with sutures further demonstrated an intense inflammatory response adjacent to the sutures and a tendency of epidermal cells to grow down the line of the incision and the suture tract into the dermis, forming unsightly needle puncture marks.[7] The localized inflammation and formation of epidermal suture-line sinus tracts associated with suturing was eliminated by using tape to close wounds.[8] Also, although sutured wounds seemed to be stronger on the fifth postoperative day, with less tendency to split open, by the tenth postoperative day, the tensile strength of the taped wounds was equivalent to that of sutured wounds.[8]

In a study[9] of 350 skin lesions closed with nylon sutures or tape (Steri-Strips;

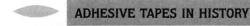 **ADHESIVE TAPES IN HISTORY**

Use of some form of tape to close wounds dates back to around 2500 BC and the ancient Egyptian civilization, where tape was used to close gaping eyebrow wounds.[1] In the 16th century, Ambroise Paré devised a method by which strips of linen were pasted to the skin edges and subsequently stitched together to avoid the unsightly stitch marks that were often noted after direct suturing of wounds.[2] A similar method was described by Lorenz Heister nearly a century later. In the 19th century, when wound infections were common and stitches could not always be trusted to hold wounds together, use of adhesive tapes became even more popular. Despite growing evidence over the past century regarding the potential advantages of surgical tapes for wound closure, they have not received widespread acceptance, largely as a result of their tendency to prematurely fall off.

3M Co., St. Paul, MN), wound closure with adhesive tape resulted in a larger proportion of cosmetically good scars than wound closure with sutures. Ferris and Henry[10] studied 287 patients with abdominal surgical wounds and also found better cosmetic results with tape closure, largely because of a reduction in the proportion of patients with scar widening and suture mark cross-hatching.

In another study[11] of 428 abdominal incisions closed with tape or suture, sutured wounds had a higher rate of infection and similar cosmetic outcome as taped wounds. Although most short-term studies comparing the cosmetic outcome of taped and sutured wounds favor taped wounds, longer-term studies fail to demonstrate significant differences in scar appearance.[12] For exam-

TABLE 7–1. ADVANTAGES AND DISADVANTAGES OF ADHESIVE TAPES FOR SKIN CLOSURE

Advantages

- Reduced costs
- Rapid and simple closure
- Least damage to host defenses
- No risk of needle-stick injuries
- Do not cause tissue ischemia or necrosis
- Do not require removal

Disadvantages

- Relatively poor adherence
- Easily removed by patient
- Must be kept dry
- Cannot be used over oily or hair-bearing areas

TABLE 7–2. INDICATIONS AND CONTRAINDICATIONS TO SKIN TAPING

Indications

- Linear, superficial lacerations subject to minimal tension
- Partial avulsions or flap lacerations
- Tissues with compromised vascular supply
- Fragile skin in elderly or steroid-dependent patients
- Support of wounds after removal of sutures or staples
- To facilitate closure of lacerations with tissue adhesives
- Undesirability of suture removal
- Tacking down skin grafts
- Under splints or casts

Contraindications

- Inadequate hemostasis
- Wounds subject to large tensions
- Irregular wounds
- Hair-bearing or oily areas
- Uncooperative patients
- Circumferential use around a digit

---

ple, Pederson and coworkers[12] followed 217 patients with abdominal wounds for up to 4 years after incision. Thread-thin scars were more common in taped wounds at 6 months, but the proportion of thread-thin scars was similar for taped and sutured wounds at the end of the 4-year observation period.[12]

Remarkably few studies based in emergency departments have compared sutures with tapes for laceration repair. Abramo[13] evaluated the use of adhesive tape (Steri-Strips) in 120 children with superficial and deep lacerations, mainly of the face and scalp. Whereas superficial wounds were managed entirely with tapes, deep wounds were closed with subcutaneous sutures as well as adhesive tape. The incidence of infection was less than 2 percent; at 3 months, most patients had fine, linear scars. However, no control group was included in this study, thereby limiting its usefulness. Similarly, Rothnie and Taylor[14] reported that most of 157 traumatic lacerations healed with satisfactory results. These wounds were located mostly on the upper extremities. Again, no control group was included for comparison.

Adhesive tapes have also been studied for closing problematic wounds such as pretibial and flap lacerations. Pretibial lacerations are often slow to heal, particularly in elderly patients who have fragile, parchment-like skin that may be torn by sutures. In a study of 76 patients with pretibial lacerations and flap lacerations, Sutton and Pritty[15] found that tapes appeared to be associated with reduced necrosis and more rapid healing than sutures. Others have also noted that adhesive tapes are preferred for the primary closure of such wounds, particularly in elderly patients.[16]

THE MECHANICAL PROPERTIES OF ADHESIVE TAPES

Surgical tapes are composed of a tape backing and an adhesive compound. Although the adhesive chemical provides the substrate for the adhesion at the wound–tape interface, the backing distributes the tension encountered in one area of the wound over the entire surface of the tape. Currently available adhesive tapes differ in their porosity, shear adhesion, flexibility, breaking strength, and elasticity (Table 7–3). Of these properties, tape shear adhesion (i.e., the ability of the tape to adhere securely to the skin) is probably the most important because it is necessary to maintain apposition of the wound edges.

MECHANICAL PERFORMANCE

The mechanical performance of a variety of commercially available adhesive tapes has been systematically evaluated by several investigators.[17–20] Although the breaking strength of Steri-Strips, a nonwoven, microporous, reinforced tape, was significantly greater than that of either Shur-Strip (Deknatel Inc., Floral Park, NY), a nonwoven, microporous tape, or Clearon (Ethicon Inc, Somerville, NJ), a synthetic plastic tape that contains longitudinal parallel serrations, Shur-Strips underwent significantly more elongation than did the other tapes and had the greatest air porosity.[17] Based on these characteristics, Rodeheaver and colleagues[17] originally recommended Shur-Strip for wound closure. Later, the same group evaluated a newer tape, Proxi-Strip (Ethicon, Inc., Somerville, NJ), and found it to be even better suited owing to its greater

TABLE 7–3. CHARACTERISTICS OF VARIOUS ADHESIVE TAPES

Product	Adhesion (alone)	Adhesion (with Adjuncts)	Air Porosity	Breaking Strength	Elongation at Breakage
Proxi-Strip*	+++	+++	+++	++	+++
Steri-Strip[†]	+	++	+	+++	+
Shur-Strip[‡]	+	++	+++	+	+++
Clearon*	+	+	+	+	+
Coverstrip[§]	+	+	UA	UA	UA
Coverstrip II[§]	++	++	UA	UA	UA
Suture-Strip[¶]	+	+++	UA	UA	UA

*Ethicon Inc., Somerville, NJ; Clearon no longer available.
[†]3M Co., St Paul, MN.
[‡]Shur Medical Corporation, Beavorton, OR. No longer available.
[§]Beirsdorf Inc., South Norwalk, CT.
[¶]Genetic Laboratories Inc, St Paul, MN.
+++ = excellent; ++ = fair to good; + = poor to fair; UA = unavailable.

level of shear adherence to the skin, air porosity, and antistatic properties that minimized the tendency of the tape strips to curl up.[18]

ADHESIVENESS

Application of tincture of benzoin to the skin edges enhanced the immediate level of adhesion of Proxi-Strip to skin, but it had little effect on the adhesiveness after the first 24 hours. From the standpoint of duration of adhesiveness, Koehn[19] found Steri-Strips superior to Clearon for wound closure. In his study of 20 volunteers, Steri-Strips remained on the skin 2.5 times longer than Clearon. Interestingly, in this study, various methods of preparing the skin before application of the adhesive strips (e.g., cleansing with alcohol or acetone or applying tincture of benzoin) had no effect on the duration of adhesion of either of the tapes.[19]

More recently, Moy and Quan[20] evaluated seven brands of wound closure tape with and without the addition of Mastisol, a liquid resin containing gum mastik. Steri-Strips with Mastisol had the longest time of adhesiveness, and the application of Mastisol markedly increased the adhesiveness of all seven tapes evaluated. However, only Proxi-Strip and Coverstrip II (Beirsdorf Inc., South Norwalk, CT) demonstrated any significant adhesiveness without Mastisol.[20] When compared with tincture of benzoin, Mastisol has been shown to markedly improve adhesive strength.[21]

Whichever adhesive adjunct is selected, care must be taken to avoid introducing the adjunct into the wound itself. In a study of five commercially available adhesive adjuncts, Panek and coworkers[22] found that all adhesive adjuncts significantly impaired the resistance of the taped wound to infection when they were introduced into the wound itself. A study by Edlich and Kuphal[23] demonstrated that the tendency of tapes to dislodge is also related to the type of solution used to prepare the skin. They found that the adhesiveness of the tapes was greater when the skin was prepped with hexachlorophene (pHisoHex) or a povidone-iodine preparation (Betadine) than when ethyl alcohol or benzal-konium chloride was used.

APPLICATION

Because adhesive tapes can be applied painlessly without anesthesia, there may be a temptation to avoid necessary wound preparation steps such as irrigation or wound débridement. Avoid giving in to this temptation. All wounds should be prepped following the basic principles noted in Chapter 3, even if a local anesthetic agent must be injected. Hemostasis should be achieved, and the wound edges should be completely dry before the tape strips are applied.

Tincture of benzoin (or better yet, Mastisol) should be applied to the wound edges, taking care to avoid accidental spillage into the wound. Brushing the wound edges with a cotton-tipped swab soaked in the adhesive solution is a good method. If benzoin is used, allow it to dry for 20 to 30 seconds before taping to increase the adhesiveness.

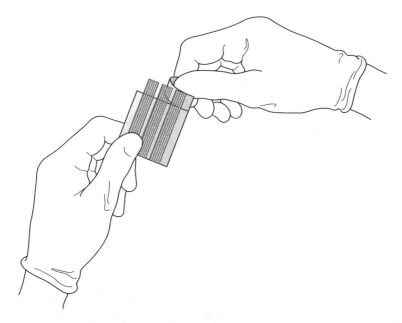

FIG. 7–1. After cutting the tape to the appropriate length. the perforated end tab is removed.

   Most tapes come in sterile packets that contain two sheets of paper backing, each with five or six strips. To facilitate handling, cut the tapes while they're still on the paper backing. Usually a length of 4 to 6 cm is adequate. After removing the perforated end of the paper backing (Fig. 7–1), individual tape strips are carefully removed from the backing with a forceps (Fig. 7–2) and

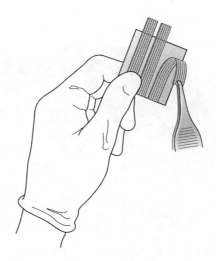

FIG. 7–2. Individual tapes are carefully removed with forceps.

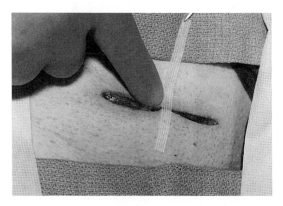

FIG. 7–3. The tape is placed on one side of the wound at its midpoint while grasping it with forceps in the dominant hand. The opposite wound edge is then gently apposed by pushing with a finger of the nondominant hand.

applied to one edge of the laceration at its midpoint, with the forceps held in the dominant hand (Fig. 7–3). The other wound edge should then be apposed by pushing with the nondominant hand, using a finger or forceps. (Using forceps is more uncomfortable and is reserved for wounds that are already anesthetized.) **The wound edges should not be apposed by pulling on the free end of the tape.** Doing so may result in unequal distribution of skin tensions; then the tape may cause erythema or even blistering of the skin. Additional strips are then placed perpendicular to the laceration on either side of the original tape, bisecting the remaining open wound with each strip until the space between tapes is no more than about 2 to 5 mm (Fig. 7–4). **To reduce the possibility of skin blistering or premature dislodgement, additional strips are then placed over the ends of the other strips, parallel to the laceration (Fig. 7–5).**

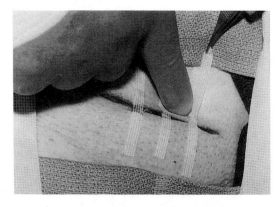

FIG. 7–4. The remaining open sections of the wound are bisected by additional tape strips until the strips are within 2 to 5 mm of each other.

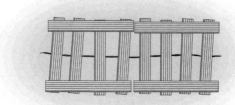

FIG. 7–5. The tape strips that were placed perpendicular to the wound are secured by placing additional strips of tape parallel to the wound at the edges of the perpendicular strips.

ADHESIVE TAPE CARE AND REMOVAL

The tapes should be left in place as long as possible, at least for the same amount of time that sutures would be left before removal. Some clinicians give patients any remaining strips of tape left from the packet and allow self-application in the event of premature dislodgement. To prevent the tapes from prematurely coming loose, warn patients to keep them as dry as possible and not to cover them with ointments. Showering is permitted, but patients should make an effort to keep the wound area dry. Patients may cover their wounds and tape with a nonadherent dressing.

REFERENCES

1. Majno, G: The Healing Hand, Man and Wound in the Ancient World. Harvard University Press, Cambridge, 1977.
2. Van Gulik, TM: The dry suture, forerunner of surgical adhesive tape. Nether J Surg 40:55–56, 1988.
3. DuMortier, JJ: The resistance of healing wounds to infection. Surg Gynecol Obstet 56:762–766, 1933.
4. Carpendale, MTF, and Sereda, W: The role of percutaneous suture and surgical wound infection. Surgery 58:672–677, 1965.
5. Edlich, RF, Rodeheaver, G, Kuphal, J, et al: Technique of closure: Contaminated wounds. JACEP 3:375–381, 1974.
6. Shauerhamer, RA, Edlich, RF, Panek, P, et al: Studies in the management of the contaminated wound. VII. Susceptibility of surgical wounds to postoperative surface contamination. Am J Surg 122:74–77, 1971.
7. Gillman, T, Penn, J, Bronks, D, et al: Re-examination of certain aspects of histogenesis of healing of cutaneous wounds: preliminary report. Br J Surg 43:141–153, 1955.
8. Gillman, T, Penn, J, Bronks, D, et al: Closure of wounds and incisions with adhesive tape. Lancet Nov 5, 945–946, 1955.
9. Depaulis, J: A critical study of causes of the problems encountered in a series of 350 skin incisions closed by means of adhesive strips. Am J Surg 113:469–471, 1967.
10. Ferris, AA, and Henry, FE: A comparative study of sutureless and suture wound closure. J Am Osteopath Assoc 65:1082–1085, 1966.

11. Conolly, WB, Hunt, TK, Zederfeldt, B, et al: Clinical comparison of surgical wounds closed by suture and adhesive tape. Am J Surg 117:318–322, 1969.
12. Pedersen, VM, Struckmann, JR, Kjaergard, HK, et al: Late cosmetic results of wound closure: strips versus suture. Neth J Surg 39:149–150, 1987.
13. Abramo, AA: Recent results with sutureless wound closure in children. Am J Dis Child 110:42–45, 1965.
14. Rothnie, NG, and Taylor, GW: Sutureless skin closure. A clinical trial. Br Med J 5364:1027–1030, 1963.
15. Sutton, R, and Pritty P: Use of sutures or adhesive tapes for primary closure of pretibial lacerations. Br Med J 290:1627, 1985.
16. Crawford, BS, and Gipson, M: The conservative management of pretibial lacerations in elderly patients. Br J Plast Surg 30:174–176, 1977.
17. Rodeheaver, GT, Halverson, JM, and Edlich, RF: Mechanical performance of wound closure tapes. Ann Emerg Med 12:203–206, 1983.
18. Edlich, RF, Spengler, MD, Morgan, RF, et al: Modern concept for a new, improved microporous skin-closure tape. JBCR 9:532–537, 1988.
19. Koehn, GG: A comparison of the duration of adhesion of Steri-Strips and Clearon. Cutis 26:620–621, 1980.
20. Moy, RL, and Quan, MB: An evaluation of wound closure tapes. J Dermatol Surg Oncol 16:721–723, 1990.
21. Mikhail, GR, Selak, L, and Salo, S: Reinforcement of surgical adhesive strips. J Dermatol Surg Oncol 12:904–906, 1986.
22. Panek, PH, Prusak, MP, Bolt, D, et al: Potentiation of wound infection by adhesive adjuncts. Am Surg 38:343–345, 1972.
23. Edlich, RF, and Kuphal, JE: Bioengineering analysis of sutureless wound closure. Intern Surg 58:246–248, 1973.

ADAM J. SINGER, MD

CHAPTER

8

Surgical Staples

The major advantages of surgical stapling include its ease of use, rapidity, cost effectiveness, and minimal damage to host defenses. It also promotes wound edge eversion, is less likely than sutures to strangulate tissues because each staple forms only an incomplete loop, and rarely leaves residual cross-hatch marks.[1] **Because the pain of applying one, two, or three staples may be less than the pain of injecting a local anesthetic agent,[2] the use of topical anesthetic agents alone may be appropriate for short lacerations. However, staple removal is more painful than removal of sutures.[3]**

Staples are ideal for closing scalp wounds. They are also very useful with linear lacerations of the torso and extremities, especially if they are relatively long. The cosmetic results achieved after repair of scalp lacerations with staples are better than those with sutures.[14] Staples may also be easier to find and remove in the scalp than sutures. Nevertheless, for meticulous tissue re-approximation, conventional suturing is probably the best option. **As a result, staples are not recommended for facial wounds.** Staples may also interfere with old-generation computed tomography (CT) scanning[16] or magnetic resonance imaging (MRI).

STUDIES AND SCIENTIFIC EVIDENCE SUPPORTING THE USE OF STAPLES

Many animal and human studies suggest that staples are comparable to sutures for the closure of most simple wounds. In animal models, although stapled and sutured wounds have similar histological and mechanical characteristics,[17] repair of contaminated wounds with staples results in lower infection rates than those repaired with sutures.[18] Although automatic stapling devices have long been used in operating rooms, few studies based in emergency departments have been reported.

THE HISTORY OF SURGICAL STAPLES

The concept of using mechanical devices to hold wound edges together is not new. The ancient Hindus used ant mandibles to keep wound edges together.[4] The first useful stapling device was developed by a Hungarian named de Petz in 1924, but its major development is attributed to the Russians.[5] Introduction of the surgical stapler in the United States by Ravitz in 1974 was followed by its adoption in a variety of surgical and medical specialties, including gastrointestinal and thoracic surgery,[5] plastic surgery,[6,7] orthopedic surgery,[8] gynecology,[9] dermatology,[10] and emergency medicine.[2,3,11–15]

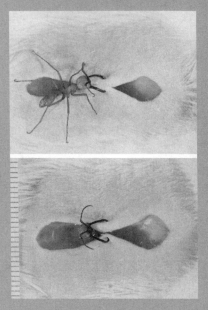

The jaws of an ant are used to hold the edges of a wound together before (upper) and after (lower) the body of the ant is twisted off. (From Majno G. The Healing Hand: Man and Wound in the Ancient World. Harvard University Press, Cambridge, Mass., 1975, with permission.)

George and Simpson[3] compared stapling with suturing in 74 patients with lacerations of the head, neck, and extremities and found stapling to be four times as fast. There was no difference between the two closure methods in respect to comfort, infection, and scar cosmesis. However, staple removal was more uncomfortable than suture removal. Similarly, Brickman and Lambert[12] evaluated skin staples in 87 lacerations to the scalp, trunk, and extremities. Skin stapling was found to be easier, quicker, and lower in cost than suture repair, without compromising wound healing or cosmetic results. Orlinsky and colleagues[13] compared the efficiency and cost of repair with staples versus sutures in 141 patients with trunk, scalp, and extremity lacerations and found that stapling was considerably faster and less expensive. MacGregor and coworkers[2] compared sutures with staples in 100 consecutive lacerations and found that the acceptability of stapling and suturing was similar for both staff and patients. Most recently, Kanegaye and associates[15] compared the total cost and physician time requirements for suture and staple repair of 88 pediatric scalp lacerations. Stapling resulted in shorter wound closure times and shorter overall times for wound care. Staple repair was also less expensive in terms of equipment ($12.55 vs. $17.59) and in terms of total cost based on equipment and physician time ($23.55 vs. $38.51). No cosmetic or infectious complications were noted in either group. These authors also found that physicians were able to perform wound repair without injecting any anesthetic agent in half the patients.

TECHNICAL ASPECTS OF SKIN STAPLING

A variety of stapling devices are commercially available for wound closure (Fig. 8–1). With all devices, the staple creates an incomplete rectangle: the legs of the staple extend into the skin, and the cross-limb lies on the skin surface

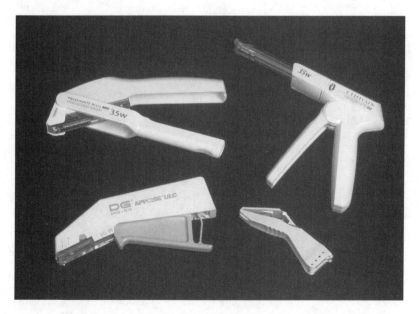

FIG. 8–1. Examples of staplers used to close skin. *(Top left)* Proximate Plus MD (Ethicon Endo-Surgery, Inc., Cincinnati, Ohio). *(Top right)* Proximate RH (Ethicon Endo-Surgery, Inc., Cincinnati, Ohio). *(Bottom left)* Appose ULC (Davis + Geck). *(Bottom right)* Precise (3M Health Care, St. Paul, Minn.).

TABLE 8–1. CHARACTERISTICS OF VARIOUS STAPLERS

Type of Stapler	Features	Benefits
Proximate RH*	Rectangular head	Minimizes staple rotation
	Head rotates 360°, cartridge is clear	Improved visibility and access
	Staples coated with Krytox	Easy staple extraction
	Pistol grip handle	Comfortable to use
Proximate PX*	Ergonomic pistol grip	Comfortable to use
	Positive ratchet mechanism	Easy staple placement
	Staples coated with Krytox	Easy staple extraction
Proximate Plus MD*	Improved kick off-spring design	Multidirectional release
	Ergonomic design	Comfortable for smaller hands
	Alignment indicator	Improves visibility
	Staples coated with Krytox	Easy staple extraction
3M Multi-shot disposable skin stapler system[†]	Small size with forceps actuation style	Allows versatile use in recessed areas
	Automatic staple release	Eliminates staple hang-ups
	Optimal preview staple position	Excellent visibility of staple at placement
	Multiple staple counts available	May save costs when small number of staples required
	Arcuate staple has similar gather as suture	Reduces staple burying and cross-hatching
	Staple has curved legs	Leaves space between skin and staple making removal easier
3M vista disposable skin stapler[†]	Angled head	Improved visualization of staple placement
	Lever action	Reduced learning curve
	Sleek handle design	Fits wide range of hand sizes
	Flexible placement angle	Allows choice in staple placement depths
	Automatic staple release lifts off in any direction	Eliminates staple hang-ups
3M PGX disposable skin stapler[†]	Slim design	Excellent visibility of staple placement
	Lightweight	Minimizes user fatigue
	Flexible placement angle	Allows choice in staple placement depth
	Ergonomically designed grip	Fits multiple hand sizes
	Automatic staple release lifts off in any direction	Eliminates staple hang-ups
Premium Plus[‡]	Head rotates 360°	Improved access
	Pistol grip	Comfortable to use
	45° angle of deployment	

TABLE 8–1. CHARACTERISTICS OF VARIOUS STAPLERS (Continued)

Type of Stapler	Features	Benefits
Premium[‡]	Head rotates 360° Pistol grip 45° angle of deployment Reusable and reloadable	Improved access Comfortable to use
Royal[‡]	Inline handle Nonrotating head 45° angle of deployment	Top span of staple floats to enhance cosmesis
Signet[‡]	Inline handle Nonrotating head 45° angle of deployment	Top span of staple floats to enhance cosmesis
Concord[‡]	Inline handle Nonrotating head 45° angle of deployment	Heavy gauge, exaggerated rectangle staple for orthopedic applications
Appose[‡]	Inline handle Nonrotating head 45° angle of deployment	Heavy gauge, exaggerated rectangle staple for orthopedic applications

*Ethicon Inc., Somerville, N.J.
[†]3M Co., St Paul, Minn.
[‡]US Surgical, Norwalk, CT.

across the wound. Although there is no clinical evidence that any particular stapler device is better than any other one, their mechanical performance varies. The stapler devices may differ in handling characteristics, maximal angle of visual access, the angle at which the staples enter tissues, the ease of positioning, and the pre-cocking mechanism (Table 8–1).[18] According to Johnson and colleagues,[18] the stapler device should allow the practitioner to optimally view the staple as it is placed in the skin. This is achieved by maximizing the angle at which the staple can be viewed during its insertion. The angle at which the staple enters the skin is also thought to be important because insertion of the staple perpendicular to the surface of the skin results in deep penetration that increases the likelihood of tissue strangulation and permanent cross-hatching of the wound. The ability of the stapler end to swivel allows the head to be adjusted for use in deep recesses. Finally, the presence of a pre-cocking mechanism allows the practitioner to maintain constant control while stapling the skin.

Before inserting staples, it is important to line up the wound edges with the centerline indicator on the head of the stapler to make sure that the legs of the staple will enter the skin at equal distances on either side of the wound edge (Fig. 8–2). Using forceps may help evert the wound edges, but it usually requires an assistant (Fig. 8–3). **Before squeezing the trigger, care should be taken to avoid excessive depression of the skin.** After the staple is inserted, a slight backward pull allows disengagement of the stapling instrument from the staple. In the case of long incisions requiring 10 or more

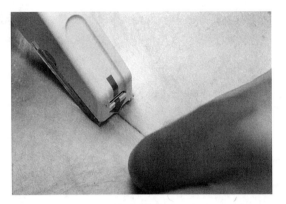

FIG. 8–2. The centerline indicator of the stapler is lined up to the wound to ensure equal bites of either side of the wound.

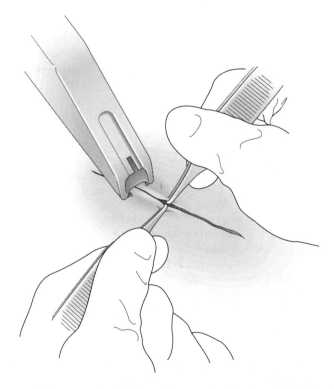

FIG. 8–3. Wound closure can be facilitated by everting the wound edges with forceps or fingers.

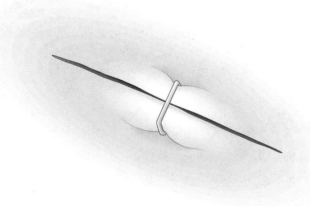

FIG. 8–4. With long lacerations, the first staple is placed in the center of the wound.

staples, it is helpful to bisect the wound into two shorter lacerations by placing the first staple in the center of the laceration (Fig. 8–4). The rest of the staples are then placed by sequentially bisecting the remaining segments of the wound.

ADVANTAGES AND DISADVANTAGES OF STAPLING

The greatest advantage of skin stapling over all other methods of wound closure is its rapidity (Table 8–2). This may be particularly important with unstable or uncooperative patients. The ability to close wounds rapidly with staples may also be very useful in situations that involve mass casualties.[3]

Skin staplers have been shown to be more cost effective when compared with sutures, especially when using staplers that contain fewer staples, such as 15 staples.[13] Because most lacerations require considerably fewer than 15 staples or sutures, use of staplers may be particularly cost effective in emergency departments and outpatient settings. The ability of staples to cause wound edge eversion is particularly valuable for elderly patients with lax skin. Staples are usually easier to find and remove in scalp wounds than are sutures. Finally, the risk of accidental needle-stick injuries is considerably less with staples than with sutures.[19]

The greatest disadvantage of skin stapling is the inability to ensure meticulous wound closure.[20] As a result, the use of skin stapling should be limited to linear lacerations not involving the face. Other disadvantages of staples are the increased discomfort during removal, the tendency to interfere with older imaging studies (e.g., head CT), and the fact that they may be very uncomfortable in body creases (e.g., groin, axilla) or over unevenly contoured skin surfaces.

TABLE 8–2. ADVANTAGES AND DISADVANTAGES OF STAPLES FOR
         SKIN CLOSURE

Advantages of Staples

- Reduced costs
- Rapid closure (appropriate for mass casualties and uncooperative or unstable patients)
- Minimal damage to host defenses
- Reduced risk of needle-stick injuries
- Provides eversion of wound edges (particularly valuable in elderly patients with lax skin)
- Easy to find among scalp hair and does not require hair clipping

Disadvantages of Staples

- Interferences with CT scans
- Discomfort during removal
- Less meticulous closure
- Uncomfortable in body creases (e.g., groin, axilla) or over uneven surfaces

INDICATIONS AND CONTRAINDICATIONS TO STAPLING

Wound closure with staples is indicated for scalp lacerations that do not require extensive hemostasis and do not involve tears in the underlying fronto-occipital aponeurosis (galea). They are also indicated for linear nonfacial lacerations caused by shear forces (e.g., sharp objects) (Table 8–3).

Skin closure with staples should not be performed if hemostasis is inadequate. Staples should also be avoided in wounds that require fine closure (e.g., facial or stellate wounds). Wounds subject to high static or dynamic ten-

TABLE 8–3. INDICATIONS AND CONTRAINDICATIONS TO SKIN STAPLING

Indications

- Scalp lacerations not requiring hemostasis or galeal repair
- Linear nonfacial lacerations caused by shear forces (e.g., sharp objects)

Contraindications

- Inadequate hemostasis
- Before CT scanning
- Not suitable when fine closure is required (e.g., facial lacerations)
- Wound subject to high tension (requires deep sutures)

sions should not be closed with staples unless underlying deep sutures are placed first.

AFTERCARE OF STAPLES

Skin staples should be removed at the same times that sutures would be removed, based on wound location and tension. For scalp wounds, staples should be removed on the seventh day after insertion. Staples should be removed from trunk and extremity wounds between days 10 and 14. Wounds closed with staples may be covered with a topical antibiotic cream or ointment as well as a dry dressing. With scalp wounds, it is often difficult to secure a dressing, and the topical antibiotic agent can be used alone. Patients may bathe or shower the next day, but they should avoid prolonged exposure to moisture. After gently washing the wound, the topical antibiotic agent should be reapplied. When staples are used in the scalp, patients should be advised to use extreme care when combing or brushing their hair.

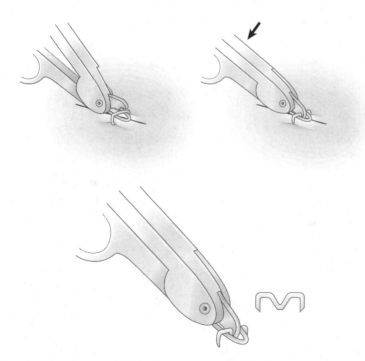

FIG. 8–5. Staple removal. The lower jaws of the staple remover are placed under the staple cross bar and the upper jaw is then compressed against the staple.

Removal of staples should be performed with a specially designed, single-handed, disposable staple remover (Fig. 8–5). The bottom double prongs should be gently placed between the staple and the underlying skin. The lever of the staple remover is then depressed slowly, lowering the single top prong. This maneuver bends the staple, releasing it from the skin.

REFERENCES

1. Edlich, RF, Becker, DG, Thacker JG, et al: Scientific basis for selecting staple and tape skin closures (review) Clin Plast Surg 17:571–578, 1990.
2. MacGregor, FB, McCombe, AW, King, PM, et al: Skin stapling of wounds in the accident department. Injury 20:347–348, 1989.
3. George, TK, and Simpson, DC: Skin wound closure with staples in the accident and emergency department. J R Coll Surg Edinb 30:54–56, 1985.
4. Majno, G: The Healing Hand, Man and Wound in the Ancient World. Harvard University Press, Cambridge, 1977, p 14.
5. Steichen, FM, and Ravitch, MM: Mechanical sutures in surgery. Br J Surg 60:191–197, 1973.
6. Ranaboldo, CJ, and Rowe-Jones, DC: Closure of laparotomy wounds: Skin staples versus sutures. Br J Surg 79:1172–1173, 1992.
7. Jones, KC, Himel, HN, Towler, MA, et al: New advances in automatic disposable rotating cartridge skin staplers. Burns 19:159–165, 1993.
8. Coupland, RM: Sutures versus staples in skin flap operations. Ann Roy Coll Surg 68:2–4, 1986.
9. Stockley, I, and Elson, RA: Skin closure using staples and nylon sutures: A comparison of results. Ann Roy Coll Surg 69:76–78, 1987.
10. Hoskin, IA, Ordorica, SA, Frieden, FJ, et al: Performance of cesarian section using absorbable staples. Surg Gynecol Obstetr 172:108–112, 1991.
11. Stegmaier, OC: Use of the skin stapler in dermatologic surgery. Am Acad Dermatol 6:305–309, 1982.
12. Brickman, KR, and Lambert, RW: Evaluation of skin stapling for wound closure in the emergency department. Ann Emerg Med 18:1122–1125, 1989.
13. Orlinsky, M, Goldberg, RM, Chan, L, et al: Cost analysis of stapling versus suturing for skin closure. Am J Emerg Med 13:77–81, 1995.
14. Hollander, JE, Giarrusso, E, and Singer, AJ: Comparison of staples and sutures for closure of scalp lacerations. Acad Emerg Med 4:460–461, 1997.
15. Kanegaye, JT, Vance, CW, Chan, L, et al: Comparison of skin stapling devices and standard sutures for pediatric scalp lacerations: A randomized study of cost and time benefits. Pediatrics 130:808–813, 1997.
16. Von Hoist, H, Bergstrom, M, and Moller, A: Titanium clips in neurosurgery for the elimination of artifacts in computerized tomography (CT). Acta Neurochir 38:101–109, 1977.
17. Roth, JH, and Windle, BH: Staple versus suture closure of skin incisions in a pig model. Can J Surg 31:19–20, 1988.
18. Johnson, A, Rodeheaver, GT, Durand, LS, et al: Automatic disposable stapling devices for wound closure. Ann Emerg Med 10:631–635, 1981.
19. Ritchie, AJ, and Rocke, LG: Staples versus sutures in the closure of scalp wounds, a prospective double blind randomized trial. Injury 20:217–218, 1989.
20. Becker, DW: Staple gun in plastic surgery (letter). Ann Plast Surgery 1:523, 1978.

ADAM J. SINGER, MD
JAMES V. QUINN, MD

CHAPTER

9

Tissue Adhesives

Several types of substances have been used in the body as tissue adhesives. These include the cyanoacrylates, methacrylates (bone glue), protein polymers, marine sealants, and fibrin sealants. In general, only two—the cyanoacrylates and fibrin sealants—have been used to close cutaneous wounds. However, the tensile strength of the fibrin sealants is low, so they are not currently recommended for the closure of traumatic wounds.[1]

STRUCTURE AND PROPERTIES OF THE CYANOACRYLATE ADHESIVES

The cyanoacrylate adhesives are synthetic liquid monomers that polymerize in the presence of basic substances to form strong bonds. First synthesized in 1949, the cyanoacrylate adhesives were evaluated clinically for wound closure 10 years later.[2] Over the past 50 years, they have enjoyed popularity as industrial and household adhesives, but not until recently have medical formulations made them popular for medical use. When used for wound closure, they are applied topically and form a bond over apposed wound edges. They usually slough off spontaneously within 5 to 10 days as the wound re-epithelializes.

The characteristics of the cyanoacrylate adhesives are determined by many factors, including the manufacturing process and the length of the alkyl or carbon side chains. The degradation products formaldehyde and cyanoacetate are both toxic to tissue and may contribute to the toxicity of these compounds.[3] Although the short-chain derivatives (e.g., methyl or ethyl cyanoacrylate) have been shown to be toxic,[4,5] the longer-chain derivatives (e.g., the butyl and octyl cyanoacrylates) are safe. In general, the shorter the alkyl side chains, the faster polymerization and degradation occur.[5]

There is negligible absorption of the cyanoacrylates when they are applied topically. The cyanoacrylates used as tissue adhesives take 6 to 9 months to degrade, by which time they have sloughed off. Medical-grade cyanoacrylate adhesives are not associated with any major toxicity or carcinogenicity.[6]

Both *in vitro* and *in vivo* models have demonstrated that the cyanoacrylate adhesives have substantial antibacterial properties for gram-positive microorganisms.[7,8] In animal models of lacerations contaminated with *Staphylococcus aureus*, the ones closed with topical tissue adhesives had fewer wound infections than those closed with sutures.[9]

Immediately after closure, the wound breaking strength of butylcyanoacrylate is less than that of a 5-0 suture. By 7 days after closure, however, the breaking strengths are similar.[10] Another study[11] showed that the breaking strength of the newer octylcyanoacrylate is three to four times greater than that of butylcyanoacrylate and is stronger than 6-0 sutures.

CLINICAL EXPERIENCE WITH THE CYANOACRYLATE ADHESIVES

Butylcyanoacrylate adhesives have been available in Europe, Israel, and Canada for several decades. They have been used successfully for the closure of traumatic lacerations and surgical incisions. The first observational report on the use of butylcyanoacrylate Histoacryl Blue (B. Braun, Melsungen AG, Melsungen, Germany) included more than 1500 children with lacerations of the scalp, face, and limbs. Follow-up methods were not detailed in the report, but only 28 children developed wound infections, and only 10 required sutures for wound dehiscence.[12]

Butylcyanoacrylate adhesives have also been used successfully for the closure of wounds resulting from various plastic and reconstructive surgeries, general surgery, urologic surgery, and otolaryngologic surgery and for application of split-thickness skin grafts.[13–15] Only recently have the cyanoacrylate adhesives been evaluated in well-designed clinical trials for wound closure. In a study[16] of 81 small facial lacerations in children presenting to the emergency department, use of butylcyanoacrylate resulted in scars comparable to those from standard 5-0 or 6-0 sutures. Application of butylcyanoacrylate was also found to be more rapid and cost effective than suturing.

A significant advance in the field of tissue adhesives was made with the development of 2-octyl-cyanoacrylate, marketed as Dermabond (Ethicon Inc., Somerville, N.J.). This tissue adhesive forms a transparent and flexible bond, unlike the opaque and brittle bond formed by the current butylcyanoacrylate adhesives. The flexibility of octylcyanoacrylate allows it to be applied over nonuniform surfaces. This flexibility also combats the topical shear forces exerted on the adhesive, reducing the risk of premature sloughing and wound dehiscence. Additionally, octylcyanoacrylate adhesive has been found to have three times the clinical breaking strength of current butylcyanoacrylate formulations, so it can be used on longer incisions and lacerations.[11] The Food and Drug Administration (FDA) recently recognized the microbial barrier function of Dermabond as long as the film remains intact.

Cosmetic results of wounds closed with cyanoacrylate adhesives are equivalent to sutures. Several clinical trials[17,18] comparing the outcome of

TABLE 9–1. COMPARISON OF TYPES OF CYANOACRYLATE ADHESIVES

	Octylcyanoacrylate Adhesives	Butylcyanoacrylate Adhesives
Number of carbons in side chain	Eight	Four
Sterility	Yes	No
Breaking strength	Moderate	Low
Flexibility	Great	Poor
Color	Transparent	Opaque
Indications	Most facial lacerations, any type of wound surface (flat or irregular contour), wounds subject to minimal or moderate tension	Short facial lacerations, flat surfaces, wounds subject to minimal tension
Microbial Barrier Function	Yes (Dermabond)	No
Length restrictions	None	Limited to short lacerations (< 4 cm)
FDA approved	Yes	No
Storage	Room temperature	Must be refrigerated

wounds closed with octylcyanoacrylate versus those closed by standard methods consistently demonstrated similar scar appearance. Wound closure with octylcyanoacrylate was more rapid and less painful than closure with sutures, yet there were no differences between the groups in wound infection and dehiscence rates. These results with octylcyanoacrylate have been echoed in other studies[19–22] that evaluated the use of this tissue adhesive for the closure of a variety of wounds resulting from head and neck surgery, general surgery, minimally invasive surgery, dermatologic surgery, or cosmetic surgery in both adults and children. A comparison of the characteristics and uses of octylcyanoacrylate and butylcyanoacrylate adhesives is presented in Table 9–1.

ADVANTAGES

In the appropriate setting, the cyanoacrylates offer several major advantages over standard wound closure techniques:

- **Tissue adhesives, which are painless to apply, are less likely to require the painful injection of local anesthetic agents.**
- **Tissue adhesives save a significant amount of time.**
- **Adhesives eliminate the need for a follow-up visit for removal of sutures**

or staples. This is a major advantage for uncooperative patients, such as small children and noncompliant patients.

- Because they do not require removal and are very comfortable for patients, the cyanoacrylate adhesives may be used under splints or casts.[23]
- **Adhesives reduce the risk to health care providers of needle-stick injuries.**
- Unlike sutures or staples, adhesives do not act as foreign bodies within the wound. This has the theoretical advantage of reducing the risk of infection.
- Adhesives do not leave suture marks.
- There is no risk of tearing fragile skin or strangulating tissue flaps with reduced vascular supply, both of which may occur with suturing.
- Overall costs are reduced by eliminating the costs of suture kits, the need for wound follow-up, and the need for suture or staple removal.[24]

DISADVANTAGES

The principal disadvantages of tissue adhesives pertain to their limited tensile strength and the likelihood that they may prematurely slough off under certain conditions. The breaking strength of octylcyanoacrylate is comparable to 5-0 or 6-0 sutures, but it is not as strong as larger sutures. The improved tensile strength of the newer octocyanoacrylate formulations is directly related to their ability to combat the shear forces exerted on the interface of the tissue adhesive and the stratum corneum. The strength of the current octylcyano-acrylate formulation is much greater than the strength of the available butyl-cyanoacrylate adhesives, largely because it is more pliable. **Nevertheless, tissue adhesives are not appropriate for closing wounds that are subject to**

TABLE 9–2. ADVANTAGES AND DISADVANTAGES OF TISSUE ADHESIVES

Advantages

- Simple
- Rapid
- Painless
- Excellent cosmetic outcome
- No need for return visit
- Cost effective
- No risk of needle-stick injuries
- Forms own protective dressing with antimicrobial barrier function
- Inherent antibacterial properties

Disadvantages

- Less tensile strength than 5-0 sutures or staples
- Less resistant to moisture than sutures or staples
- May impede healing if introduced into wound depth
- Need for proper positioning to prevent runoff

significant static or dynamic tensions (e.g., over joints) unless deep sutures, immobilization, or both are also used. They also are inappropriate for areas subject to repetitive friction or moisture. Because it is almost impossible to avoid friction and moisture on the hands and feet, tissue adhesives are not recommended for closure of wounds in these areas. The advantages and disadvantages of tissue adhesives are summarized in Table 9–2.

INDICATIONS AND CONTRAINDICATIONS

The cyanoacrylate adhesives are particularly useful for closure of noncontaminated wounds that are under minimal tension. **Tissue adhesives should be used only when the wound edges can be easily approximated.** Most wounds occur in the head and neck. These areas have low wound infection rates and low tension, making the cyanoacrylate adhesives ideally suited for closure of these lacerations. The adhesives may also be used safely over the torso and areas of the extremities that are not subject to significant tension. In areas that are subject to moderate tension, using deep sutures may allow easy approximation of skin edges and closure with tissue adhesives. **Even when deep sutures are placed, tissue adhesives should often be used because they reduce time requirements and eliminate the need for follow-up and suture removal.** Tissue adhesives may also be used over joints if they are to be splinted.[25] Tissue adhesives are also useful for closing various skin flaps, where addition of sutures may further compromise their vascular supply. Adhesives may also be used to close lacerations over fragile skin that is easily torn by sutures, such as the skin over the lower leg, especially in elderly patients.

Tissue adhesives are not currently recommended if there is an increased risk

TABLE 9–3. INDICATIONS AND CONTRAINDICATIONS FOR USING TISSUE ADHESIVES

Indications

- Closure of easily approximated lacerations and incisions
- Closure of flaps
- Closure of lacerations over fragile skin
- Attachment of skin grafts to recipient site

Contraindications

- Active infection or heavy contamination
- Mucosal surfaces and mucocutaneous borders
- Fluid-bathed surfaces
- Hair-bearing areas
- High-tension areas
- Areas subject to repetitive friction
- Allergy to the cyanoacrylates or formaldehyde

of infection or poor healing, such as in immunocompromised patients or wounds that are contaminated or poorly vascularized. It is possible, however, that future research may demonstrate their advantage over sutures for such patients and wounds. Other relative contraindications to the application of tissue adhesives include wounds involving mucosal surfaces or mucocutaneous borders, areas with dense hair, and areas routinely exposed to bodily fluids. The cyanoacrylate adhesives are contraindicated for patients with a known hypersensitivity to cyanoacrylate or formaldehyde. The indications and contraindications for use of the cyanoacrylate adhesives are summarized in Table 9–3.

APPLICATION

Application of tissue adhesives is a manual skill that is easily acquired but does require some practice and training to master control of the applicator and adhesive viscosity. Mastery of tissue adhesive use is quite rapid. A study[26] comparing the cosmetic outcome of lacerations repaired with tissue adhesives and sutures found that results were excellent regardless of how often the physician had used adhesives in the past, although all physicians in the study had some basic instruction. In contrast, 1 to 2 years of experience are required before a practitioner becomes proficient at suturing traumatic lacerations.[27]

The need for proper wound selection, evaluation, and meticulous preparation before closure with tissue adhesives is paramount.[28] **Wounds must be thoroughly cleansed and débrided in accordance with standard practice before using adhesives. The clinician must also ensure that the wound edges are tightly apposed so that the adhesive is not placed into the wound.** If adhesive is spilled into the wound itself, it impedes epithelialization of the wound edges and may result in inflammatory reactions.[29] If the clinician is not pleased with wound edge apposition, tissue adhesives should not be used. It is important to maintain proper eversion of the skin edges and precise wound approximation as the adhesive polymerizes, which may take from 30 to 60 seconds, depending on the type used.

Application of tissue adhesives requires a relatively dry surface. Hemostasis can usually be obtained by applying direct pressure over the wound with sterile gauze. Applying a 1:1000 to 1:2000 topical epinephrine solution (alone or in combination with lidocaine and tetracaine) to the wound bed may also enhance hemostasis. Use of a combined solution containing a local anesthetic as well as epinephrine (e.g., LET, a combination of lidocaine 2%, epinephrine 1:1000, and tetracaine 2%) has the advantages of combining hemostatic properties with anesthetic effects needed for exploration and irrigation when necessary. If hemostasis cannot be obtained, the wound may instead need to be closed with sutures.

Because the current adhesives are low in viscosity, runoff can be a problem. **Patient positioning is critical to reduce runoff of tissue adhesive. The patient should be positioned so that the wound surface is parallel to the floor, taking special care that any runoff does not flow in the direction of vital structures such as the eye (Fig. 9–1).** Vital structures that are adjacent to the wound should be covered with dry gauze (Fig. 9–2). Holding dry gauze

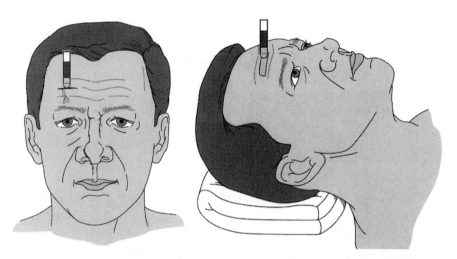

FIG. 9–1. The patient should be positioned such that the wound plane is parallel to the floor. With lacerations above the eye, the patient should be in the supine position *(Right)*, not erect *(Left)*. (From Quinn, JV: Tissue Adhesives in Wound Care. Hamilton, Ontario, BC Decker Inc, 1998, p 47, with permission.)

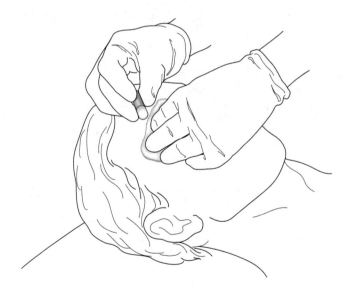

FIG. 9–2. With lacerations over the eye, the eye should be covered with dry gauze. (From Quinn, JV: Tissue Adhesives in Wound Care. Hamilton, Ontario, BC Decker Inc, 1998, p 56, with permission.)

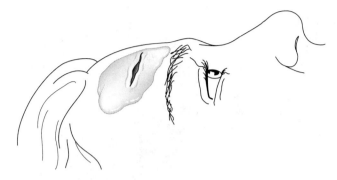

FIG. 9–3. In order to limit runoff of the adhesive, the wound may be surrounded by a rim of ointment.

in the hand that is grasping the adhesive applicator allows for rapid wiping of any adhesive that has started to run. The wound may also be surrounded by a rim of petrolatum or a topical antibiotic ointment to block adhesive runoff (Fig. 9–3). With experience, the clinician can minimize runoff by gently squeezing and releasing the pressure on the vial to control the amount of adhesive that is expressed.

A newly available chisel-shaped tip for the octylcyanoacrylate adhesives further reduces the tendency for runoff by allowing more controlled expression of the adhesive through the tip. Avoiding excessive expression of the adhesive also minimizes the chances that the practitioner's fingers will get stuck to the wound. If the practitioner thinks that his or her gloved hand has come in contact with the adhesive and fears getting stuck to the patient's skin, the other hand should be used to reinforce wound apposition while the original hand is gently pulled away from the wound.

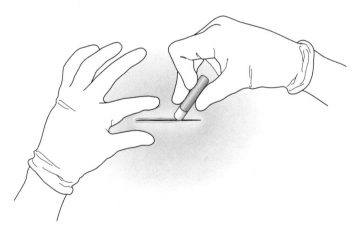

FIG. 9–4. The wound edges are held in apposition with the fingers of the nondominant hand.

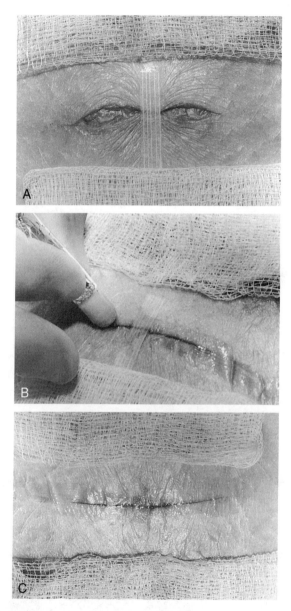

FIG. 9–5. Closing a long or complex wound. *(A)* The wound is bisected with a strip of surgical tape. *(B)* The wound limbs on either side of the tape are glued. *(C)* The tape is removed and the central portion of the wound is glued. Some practitioners prefer to leave the tape strip and apply the adhesive over it.

To avoid getting adhesive into the wound, the wound edges may be held together by one of several methods. For short, simple, linear lacerations that are under minimal tension, the wound edges may be apposed with the practitioner's fingers or delicate, atraumatic forceps (Fig. 9–4). If the wound is particularly long or complicated, an assistant can help hold the wound edges together as the adhesive polymerizes. Long lacerations or incisions or lacerations with multiple limbs may be divided into discrete segments and closed in stages (Fig. 9–5). Securing the wound at intervals with surgical tapes may make wound closure easier by ensuring proper wound apposition.

Butylcyanoacrylate adhesives such as Histoacryl Blue polymerize rapidly on contact with the skin, usually within 10 to 15 seconds. As a result, they are applied in a pattern of discrete drops along the wound surface, a technique that is similar to spot welding (Fig. 9–6). Because these adhesives tend to be brittle, they are best suited for short lacerations over relatively flat surfaces (see Table 9–1). To apply Histoacryl Blue, the tip of the vial is cut off and the adhesive is expressed either directly from the tip of the vial or through a 25-gauge needle that is attached to the hub of the vial (Fig. 9–7). The needle allows more precise application. With Indermal, another type of butylcyanoacrylate adhesive, the adhesive is expressed directly from the tip of the applicator.

Octylcyanoacrylate is supplied in a glass vial within a plastic container. The vial should be gently crushed and the adhesive expressed through the tip of the applicator (Fig. 9–8). This kind of adhesive forms a thin, flexible bond, which sets more slowly, usually within 30 to 60 seconds. This adhesive should be applied over the entire wound area with a gentle brushing

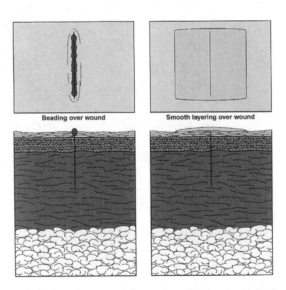

FIG. 9–6. *(Left)* With the butylcyanoacrylates, the adhesive is applied as discrete bead. *(Right)* With octylcyanoacrylate, the adhesive is applied as one continuous film across the entire wound. (From Quinn, JV: Tissue Adhesives in Wound Care. Hamilton, Ontario, BC Decker Inc, 1998, p 46, with permission.)

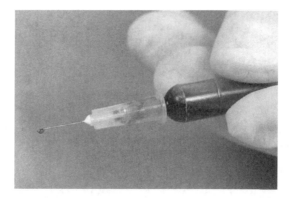

FIG. 9–7. The tip of the butylcyanoacrylate applicator is cut off and a small needle is attached to its end, allowing more precise application of the adhesive. (From Quinn JV. Tissue Adhesives in Wound Care. Hamilton, Ontario, BC Decker, 1998, p 51, with permission.)

motion parallel to the wound, including a rim of normal tissue extending 5 to 10 mm on either side of the wound (see Fig. 9–4). This increases the surface area to which the adhesive adheres. The adhesive should be distributed evenly over the surface of the wound (Fig. 9–9), taking care that no adhesive gets between the wound edges. After allowing the first layer to partially

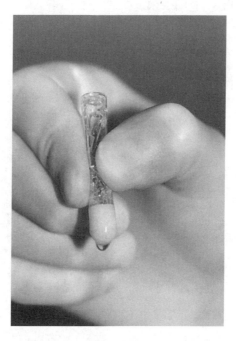

FIG. 9–8. Octylcyanoacrylate is expressed from its applicator by carefully squeezing the plastic container after the glass vial has been gently crushed.

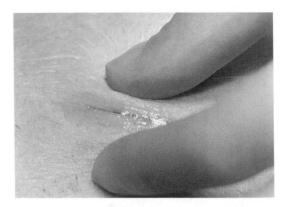

FIG. 9–9. The adhesive is applied evenly across the entire wound, including a margin of at least 5 to 10 mm on either side of the wound.

polymerize for 30 to 60 seconds, the practitioner should apply another two or three layers of adhesive, allowing 10 to 15 seconds between each application.

POTENTIAL PITFALLS

INADEQUATE WOUND PREPARATION

Proper wound selection and application technique can avoid most problems associated with the use of tissue adhesives. The major potential pitfall of using tissue adhesives is not spending enough time evaluating, selecting, and preparing wounds. All wounds should be evaluated similarly regardless of the method used for wound closure. Although anesthesia may not be required for closure, it may still be needed for wound exploration and cleansing.

RUNOFF

As already discussed, problems with runoff can be avoided in several ways. If adhesive does accidentally run into the patient's eye, the patient should widely open his or her eyelids to avoid matting of the eyelashes. Matted eyelashes should not be cut. An ophthalmic ointment, such as erythromycin or Bacitracin, should be applied to help accelerate sloughing of the adhesive, and the eye should be patched. The cyanoacrylate adhesives are not toxic to the globe and do not cause any long-term ophthalmic toxicity. A higher viscosity formulation of Dermabond is currently under investigation.

WOUND DEHISCENCE

Wound dehiscence is usually the result of improper wound selection, improper adhesive application, or both. If a wound is subject to significant static or dynamic tensions, tissue adhesives should be applied only in conjunction with deep sutures, splinting and immobilization of the affected joint, or a combination of these. Wounds that cannot be easily approximated with forceps or fingers should not be closed with tissue adhesives alone. Premature sloughing of the tissue adhesive with dehiscence may also occur with recurrent friction and exposure to moisture. If the patient will not be able to keep the wound relatively dry for at least a week, tissue adhesives should be avoided.

If wound dehiscence occurs, the wound may be closed by reapplying the tissue adhesive or by using a different technique. The choice of subsequent wound closure method should depend, in part, on the reasons for dehiscence. If high tension was the cause, for instance, deep sutures should be used.

INFECTION

Wound infections usually result from improper wound preparation or improper adhesive application. It may be tempting to close wounds with tissue adhesives without exploring, débriding, or irrigating them, but this should never be done. If tissue adhesive is improperly applied between wound edges, it not only prevents epithelialization and promotes the chance of dehiscence, but it may also increase the risk of infection by acting as a foreign body.

Table 9–4 presents a summary of potential problems associated with use of tissue adhesives and ways to avoid or manage them.

TABLE 9–4. POTENTIAL PROBLEMS WITH TISSUE ADHESIVES

Problem	Ways To Avoid the Problem
Runoff	Position patient with wound parallel to floor. Circumscribe wound with ointment.
Spillage into eyes	Cover eyes with gauze barrier. Position patient so wound is not above eye. Apply petrolatum jelly barrier before applying adhesive.
Wound dehiscence	Avoid adhesive use for high-tension wounds. Avoid frequent exposure to friction or moisture. **Use deep sutures or immobilization for high-tension wounds.**
Wound infection	**Use adhesives only for properly selected wounds (see Table 9–3).** Use proper wound preparation, including irrigation, exploration, and (when necessary) débridement. Use proper application techniques (see text).
Getting stuck to the wound	Practice expressing small amounts of adhesive and controlling runoff. Alternate the hand used to appose wound edges before complete polymerization of the adhesive.

TABLE 9–5. PATIENT INSTRUCTIONS FOR WOUND CARE AFTER APPLICATION OF TISSUE ADHESIVES

- Check your wound daily. Contact your doctor if there is significant swelling, redness, warmth, or pus.
- Return if your wound opens up. As long as it is not infected, it may be repaired again with either adhesive or sutures (stitches).
- You may cover your wound with a dry bandage.
- Do not scratch, rub, or pick at the adhesive.
- You may take a shower or a bath, but do not scrub or soak your wound.
- Do not place any adhesive tape directly on your wound.
- Do not apply any cream or ointment onto the adhesive.
- The adhesive will fall off on its own within 5 to 10 days.

WOUND AFTERCARE

Wounds should be kept clean and dry to avoid premature sloughing of the adhesive. The wound may be allowed to get wet briefly during showering or bathing, but patients should avoid scrubbing or soaking the wound. Swimming and periods of heavy perspiration may also result in premature sloughing of the adhesive.

Tissue adhesives form their own dressing. As a result, no further dressings are required. Some patients may prefer to cover their wound with a clean, dry dressing. Such coverings are permissible after the tissue adhesive has completely dried, but adhesive tape should not be applied directly to the tissue adhesive. No liquids or ointments, such as topical antibiotic agents, should be applied because they may loosen the adhesive film. A sample of patient instructions for care of wounds closed with tissue adhesives is presented in Table 9–5.

REFERENCES

1. Toriumi, DM, Lovice, D, and O'Grady, KM: Fibrin tissue adhesive in otolaryngology-head and neck surgery. J Long Term Eff Med Implants 8:143–159, 1998.
2. Coover, HN, Joyner, FB, and Sheere, NH: Chemistry and performance of cyanoacrylate adhesive. J Soc Plast Surg Eng 15:5–6, 1959.
3. Pani, KC, Gladieux, G, Brandes, G, et al: The degradation of n-butyl alpha-cyanoacrylate tissue adhesive. II. Surgery 63:481–489, 1968.
4. Kulkarni, RK, Hanks, GA, Pani, KC, et al: The in vivo metabolic degradation of poly(methyl cyanoacrylate) via thiocyanate. J Biomed Mater Res 1:11–16, 1967.
5. Leonard, F, Hodge, JW Jr, Houston, S, et al: Alpha-cyanoacrylate adhesive bond strengths with proteinaceous and non-proteinaceous substrates. J Biomed Mater Res 2:173–178, 1968.
6. Kung, H: Evaluation of the undesirable side effects of the surgical use of Histoacryl glue with special regard to possible carcinogenicity. RCC Institute for Contract Research, Basel, Switzerland. 1986 Mar, project 064315.
7. Matsumoto, T, Dobek, AS, Pani, KC, et al: Bacteriological study of cyanoacrylate tissue adhesives. Arch Surg 97:527–530, 1968.
8. Quinn, JV, Ramotar, K, and Osmond, MH: Antimicrobial effects of a new tissue adhesive. Acad Emerg Med 3:536–537, 1996.

9. Quinn, JV, Maw, JL, Ramotar, K, et al: Octylcyanoacrylate tissue adhesive wound repair versus suture wound repair in a contaminated wound model. Surgery 122:69–72, 1997.
10. Noordzij, JP, Foresman, PA, Rodeheaver, GT, et al: Tissue adhesive wound repair revisited. J Emerg Med 12:645–649, 1994.
11. Perry, LC: An evaluation of acute incisional strength with Traumaseal surgical tissue adhesive wound closure. Dimensional Analysis Systems Inc., Leonia, NJ, 1995.
12. Mizrahi, S, Bickel, A, and Ben-Layish, EB: Use of tissue adhesives in the repair of lacerations in children. J Pediatr Surg 23:312–313, 1988.
13. Keng, TM, and Bucknall, TE: A clinical trial of tissue adhesive in skin closure of groin wounds. Med J Malaysia 44:122–128, 1989.
14. Smyth, GD, and Kerr, AG: Histoacryl (butyl cyanoacrylate) as an ossicular adhesive. J Laryngol Otol 88:539–542, 1974.
15. Ousterhout, DK, Tumbusch, WT, Margetis, PM, et al: The treatment of split thickness skin graft donor sites using n-butyl and n-heptyl 2-cyanoacrylate. Br J Plast Surg 24:23–30, 1971.
16. Quinn, JV, Drzewiecki, A, Li, MM, et al: A randomized, controlled trial comparing a tissue adhesive with suturing in the repair of pediatric facial lacerations. Ann Emerg Med 22:1130–1135, 1993.
17. Quinn, JV, Wells, GA, Sutcliffe, T, et al: A randomized trial comparing octylcyanoacrylate tissue adhesive and sutures in the management of lacerations. JAMA 277:1527–1530, 1997.
18. Singer, AJ, Hollander, JE, Valentine, SM, et al: Prospective randomized controlled trial of a new tissue adhesive (2-octylcyanoacrylate) versus standard wound closure techniques for laceration repair. Acad Emerg Med 5:94–98, 1998.
19. Maw, JL, Quinn, JV, Wells, GA, et al: A prospective comparison of octylcyanoacrylate tissue adhesive and sutures for the closure of head and neck incisions. J Otolaryngol 26:26–30, 1997.
20. Toriumi, DM, O'Grady, K, Desai, D, et al: Use of octyl-2-cyanoacrylate for skin closure in facial plastic surgery. Plast Reconstr Surg 102:2209–2219, 1998.
21. Bruns, T, Robinson, B, Smith, R, et al: A new tissue adhesive for laceration repair in children. J Pediatr 32:1067–1070, 1998.
22. Singer, AJ, Quinn, JV, Clark, RE, et al: Closure of lacerations and incisions with octylcyanoacrylate: a multi-center randomized controlled trial. Surgery 131:270–276, 2002.
23. Penoff, J: Skin closure using cyanoacrylate tissue adhesives. Plast Reconstr Surg 103:730–731, 1999.
24. Osmond, MH, Klassen, TP, and Quinn, JV: Economic comparison of a tissue adhesive and suturing in the repair of pediatric facial lacerations. J Pediatr 126:892–895, 1995.
25. Saxena, AK, and Willital, GH: Octylcyanoacrylate tissue adhesive in the repair of pediatric extremity lacerations. Am Surg 65:470–472, 1999.
26. Hollander, JE, and Singer, AJ: Application of tissue adhesive: Rapid attainment of proficiency. Acad Emerg Med 5:1012–1017, 1998.
27. Singer, AJ, Hollander, JE, Valentine, SM, et al: Association of training level and short-term appearance of repaired lacerations. Acad Emerg Med 3:378–383, 1996.
28. Quinn, JV: Tissue Adhesives in Wound Care, ed 1. BC Decker Inc., Hamilton, Canada, 1998.
29. Singer, AJ, Berruti, L, McClain, SA: Comparative trial of octyl-cyanoacrylate and silver sulfadiazine for the treatment of full-thickness skin biopsies. Wound Repair and Regeneration 7:356–361, 1999.

JUDD E. HOLLANDER, MD
ADAM J. SINGER, MD

C H A P T E R

10

Selecting Sutures and Needles for Wound Closure

There are several different techniques for performing a cosmetically appealing repair of lacerated tissue. In each situation, the optimal closure technique should be based on consideration of the biological properties of the materials to be used, the anatomical configuration of the injury, and the biomechanical properties of the wound. This chapter summarizes the various suture materials and needles available for closure of traumatic lacerations and incisions.

CONSIDERATIONS IN SUTURE SELECTION

In general, the techniques of suture closure of skin can be divided into two types: percutaneous sutures and dermal (subcuticular) sutures. The wound's configuration and biomechanical properties, as well as other special circumstances, influence the selection of the technique for closure. The choice of suture materials depends on whether the wound closure occurs in one or more layers. In selecting the most appropriate sutures for each particular wound, practitioners must take into account the amount of tension on the wound, number of layers of closure, depth of suture placement, anticipated amount of edema, and anticipated timing of suture removal.

INFECTION

All sutures potentially impair the local tissue defenses that prevent infection. Needle insertion itself causes a small inflammatory response. Sutures also penetrate the intact skin, thereby providing a means for bacteria to descend to the depth of the wound. The presence of the suture material within

the wound increases the likelihood of infection. The li)
related to both the amount of suture within the tissu/
ture material used. Also, sutures that are tied too tigh
fenses, further increasing the risk of infection./
polypropylene (PP), or polybutester (PBE) sutures a.
cutaneous closure of skin wounds because these suture m
the least damage to the wound's defenses.[2]

Synthetic absorbable sutures elicit the least inflammatory response of
the absorbable sutures. Plain and chromic gut elicits a greater inflammatory response. Of the nonabsorbable sutures, nylon, PP, PBE, and polytetrafluoroethylene sutures are the least reactive.[1] Sutures made of natural fibers
potentiate infection more than any other nonabsorbable sutures; this corre-
lates with the tissue's reaction to these sutures in clean wounds.[2] Based on
clinical experience and supportive experimental studies, silk and cotton sutures should not be used in wounds that have gross bacterial contamination.
These materials should not be used for most wound closures because they
have increased inflammatory properties and do not appear to have significantly better handling characteristics than the less reactive nylon sutures.
As a result, there is no clinical role for these natural fiber sutures in wound
closure.

The physical configuration of sutures also is related to the likelihood of developing infection. **Monofilament sutures (constructed from one filament)**
have lower infection rates than multifilament sutures.[3] **Larger-diameter**
sutures are associated with greater impairment of tissue defenses; there-
fore, practitioners should generally use the smallest-diameter suture (5-0
or 6-0) with sufficient strength to maintain wound closure.

WOUND EDEMA

Any injured tissue will develop edema over 24 to 48 hours after injury. Sutures that can stretch and then return to their original length as the edema
develops and resolves possess an advantage over sutures without this ability. PBE is one such suture.[4] Nylon, PP, polyester, and silk do not stretch with
swelling. As a result, they may lacerate or necrose tissues that develop large
amounts of edema, increasing the likelihood of infection or suboptimal cosmetic result.

SUTURE REMOVAL

One of the suture characteristics to consider is the coefficient of friction. Sutures such as PBE with low coefficients of friction can be easily removed
without requiring considerable force to separate the suture from the surrounding tissue.[5] Easy removal of sutures minimizes the likelihood that sutures will break and leave residual suture within the healing laceration. For
most lacerations in which sutures are left in place for short periods, the ease
of suture removal of the less costly nylon and PP suture is quite adequate.

AILS OF SUTURE MATERIALS

he degradation properties of sutures separate them into two general categories, absorbable and nonabsorbable. Sutures that undergo rapid degradation in tissues, losing their tensile strength within 60 days, are considered absorbable sutures. Sutures that generally maintain their tensile strength for longer than 60 days are nonabsorbable sutures. It must be noted that even nonabsorbable sutures do lose some of their tensile strength during this period.[6] A distinction should be made between the rate of absorption and the rate at which the suture material loses its tensile strength. The rate of absorption is important with respect to complications such as the development of sinus tracts and granulomas. The loss of tensile strength is of greater clinical significance because the primary function of the suture is to maintain wound edge apposition during healing.

NONABSORBABLE SUTURES

Nonabsorbable sutures can be classified according to their origin as natural (e.g., silk) or synthetic (e.g., polyamides [nylon], polyesters [Dacron], polyolefins [polyethylene, PP], polytetrafluoroethylene, or PBE). Nonabsorbable sutures are also characterized by their physical configurations. Nylon, PP, PBE, polytetrafluoroethylene, and stainless steel are available as monofilament sutures. Nylon, polyester, stainless steel, silk, and cotton sutures are available as multifilament sutures. Only nylon and stainless steel sutures are available as both a monofilament and a multifilament suture. Synthetic sutures are superior to sutures derived from natural sources. Table 10–1 summarizes the characteristics and common uses of nonabsorbable sutures.

Polypropylene sutures have a low coefficient of friction that facilitates knot rundown and suture passage through the tissue.[5] They are extremely inert in tissue, and they retain their tensile strength in tissues for years. They also exhibit a lower drag coefficient in tissue than nylon sutures, making them ideal for use in continuous dermal and percutaneous suture closure (see Chapter 11). However, they stretch under high pressures, so the suture loop is widened as edema resolves. This widening may allow wound edges to separate if the sutures were placed when a large amount of edema was present. *Nylon* sutures are more pliable and easier to handle than PP sutures, but there do not appear to be proven clinical differences between nylon and PP sutures. The slightly lower propensity for erythema with PP sutures may make them the preferred sutures for patients at risk for inflammatory reactions or keloid formation.

The largest clinical difference between PP and nylon sutures might be the colors (nylon is black, and PP is blue). PBE sutures have unique performance characteristics that are advantageous. They are as strong as the other monofilament sutures, they exhibit similar degrees of elongation and have the same knotting characteristics; however, they are more flexible and elastic (i.e., they stretch). The superior elasticity allows the suture to return to its original length after the load is removed. It also decreases tension on the wound, thereby

TABLE 10–1. CHARACTERISTICS OF THE NONABSORBABLE SUTURES

Suture	Structure	Raw Material	Tensile Strength Retention *in Vivo*	Absorption Rate	Tissue Reactivity	Commom Uses
Silk	Braided	Organic protein called fibroin	Degradation of fiber results in loss of strength over many months	Nonabsorbable	Significant inflammatory reaction	Intra-oral mucosal surfaces for comfort
Nylon (Ethilon, Dermalon)	Monofilament	Polyamide polymer	Hydrolysis results in loss of strength over years	Nonabsorbable	Minimal	Soft tissue and skin reapproximation
PP (Prolene, Surgipro)	Monofilament	PP polymer	No degradation or weakening	Nonabsorbable	Least	Soft tissue and skin reapproximation
Polyester (Mersilene, Ticron)	Braided and monofilament	Polyethylene terephthalate	No degradation or weakening	Nonabsorbable	Minimal	Tendon repair using undyed (white) color
PBE (Novafil)	Monofilament	Poly (butylene) and poly (tetramethylene ether) glycol terephthalate	No degradation or weakening	Nonabsorbable	Minimal	Soft tissue approximation, easy handling and knot security

PP = polypropelene; PBE = polybutester.

101

TABLE 10–2. CHARACTERISTICS OF THE ABSORBABLE SUTURES

Suture	Types	Material	Tensile Strength Retention *in Vivo*	Absorption Rate	Tissue Reactivity	Common Uses
Surgical gut	Plain	Collagen derived from bovine intestine	Retains 50% tensile strength for 5–7 days	Absorbed by proteolytic processes in weeks	Moderate reactivity	Rarely, for intraoral wounds
Chromic gut	Chromium coating	Collagen derived from bovine intestine	Retains 50% tensile strength for 10–14 days	Absorbed by proteolytic processes in weeks	Moderate reactivity	Rarely, for subcutaneous closures and intraoral wounds
Polyglycolic acid (Dexon)	Braided	Polymer of glycolic acid	Retains 65% tensile strength at 2 weeks; 35% at 3 weeks	Completely absorbed by slow hydrolysis by 60–90 days	Minimal	Approximation of deep soft tissue structures (i.e., dermis); for ligation
Polyglactin 910 (Vicryl)	Braided	Copolymer of lactide and glycolide with polyglactin 370 and calcium stearate	Retains 75% tensile strength at 2 weeks; 50% at 3 weeks	Completely absorbed by slow hydrolysis by 56–70 days	Minimal	Approximation of deep soft tissue structures (i.e., dermis); for ligation
Polyglactin 910 (Vicryl Rapide)	Braided	Copolymer of glycolide and lactide coated with polyglactin 370 and calcium stearate	Retains 50% tensile strength for 5 days; all lost by 2 weeks	Absorbed by hydrolysis. Usually complete by 42 days	Minimal	Skin approximation when absorbable sutures used

Suture	Structure	Material	Tensile Strength	Absorption	Tissue Reaction	Use
Polyglactin 910 (Lactomer)	Braided	Copolymer of glycolide and lactide coated with caprolactone and glycolide	Retains 40% tensile strength for 3 weeks	Absorbed by hydrolysis. Usually complete by 56–70 days.	Minimal	Subcutaneous soft tissue approximation
Polydioxanone (PDS II)	Monofilament	Polyester polymer	Retains 70% strength for 2 weeks; 50% tensile strength for 4 weeks; 25% for 6 weeks	Minimal until 90 days; complete by 6 months	Minimal	Subcutaneous soft tissue approximation when more prolonged strength is needed
Poliglecaprone 25 (Monocryl)	Monofilament	Copolymer of glycolide and epsilon-caprolactine	Retains 60%–70% tensile strength for one week; 30%–40% at 2 weeks	Absorbed by hydrolysis within 3–4 months	Minimal	Subcutaneous soft tissue approximation
Glycomer 631	Monofilament	Terpolymer of glycolide, trimethylene carbonate and dioxanone	Retains 70% tensile strength 28 days; 13% at 56 days	Complete by 90–110	Slight	Subcutaneous soft tissue approximation when more prolonged strength is needed
Lactide glycolide (Panacryl)	Braided	Copolymer of lactide and glycolide	Retains 80% tensile strength at 3 months; 60% at 6 months; 20% at 1 year	Complete within 1.5–2.5 years	Minimal	Subcutaneous soft tissue approximation (e.g., fascia) when more prolonged strength is needed; excellent handling
Polyglyconate (Maxon)	Monofilament	Polyglyconate polymer	Retains 70% tensile strength 28 days; 13% at 56 days	Complete by 90–110 days	Slight	Subcutaneous soft tissue approximation when more prolonged strength is needed

reducing the tendency for hypertrophic scarring.[7] *Polyester* sutures are composed of fibers of polyester, or polyethylene terephthalate, a synthetic linear polyester. Polyester sutures are synthetic, braided sutures that last indefinitely in tissues. As a result, undyed polyester sutures, which are not likely to be visible through the skin, are primarily used for the repair of tendon lacerations.

ABSORBABLE SUTURES

Absorbable sutures (Table 10–2) are made from either natural sources (e.g., collagen) or synthetic polymers.

Natural Absorbable Sutures

The collagen sutures are derived from the submucosal or the serosal layer of bovine small intestine (gut). *Chromic gut* is more highly cross-linked than plain gut and is more resistant to absorption. Gut is resorbed via lysosomal enzymes.[8]

Natural absorbable sutures are seldom used for the repair of traumatic lacerations. They may fray during knot construction, and their tensile strength varies considerably. These sutures are used for wounds that involve mucosal surfaces subject to minimal tension (e.g., inside the mouth). Nonabsorbable synthetic sutures are preferred for most epidermal nonmucosal skin closures.

Synthetic Braided Absorbable Sutures

Synthesis of high–molecular weight polyglycolic acid and polylactic acid produces *polyglycolic acid* sutures and *polyglactin* 910 sutures. The copolymers of polyglactin 910 are prepared by polymerizing nine parts of glycolide with one part of lactide; the polyglycolic acid sutures are produced from the homopolymer. Because of the inherent rigidity of these copolymers, they are extruded into thin filaments and braided.[9] The polyglycolic acid and polyglactin 910 sutures degrade in an aqueous environment through hydrolysis of the ester linkage. *Lactomer glycolide or lactide* sutures provide a high initial tensile strength with slow, uniform degradation in tissues. The smaller filaments in this braided suture enhance tensile strength, reduce the coefficient of friction, and improve handling. The surfaces of these synthetic sutures have been coated to decrease their coefficient of friction.[9] *Panacryl* (a copolymer of lactide and glycolide) is a braided synthetic absorbable suture with excellent long-term strength retention. Its initial tensile strength is comparable to that of braided polyester nonabsorbable sutures. It maintains 80 percent of its initial tensile strength at 3 months and 60 percent for up to 6 months. A coating allows for smooth passage and reduces friction during knot construction. Panacryl is particularly useful when extended wound support is needed. It is indicated for many operative procedures, but it is usually not required for traumatic lacerations.

Synthetic Monofilament Absorbable Sutures

Polydioxanone (PDS II) is a monofilament absorbable suture[10] that is processed into small granules and extruded into monofilaments. *Glycolide trimethylene carbonate* is a linear copolymer made by reacting trimethylene carbonate and glycolide, with diethylene glycol as an initiator and stannous chloride dihydrate as the catalyst. *Polyglecaprone 25* is a synthetic absorbable suture that is one of the most pliable synthetic absorbable monofilament sutures available commercially. *Glycomer 631* is a monofilament synthetic absorbable suture that is significantly stronger than the braided synthetic absorbable suture over 4 weeks of implantation.[11] This monofilament suture also potentiates less bacterial infection than does the braided suture. The monofilament synthetic absorbable suture maintains its strength much longer *in vivo* than the braided synthetic absorbable sutures. These monofilament sutures retain approximately 70 percent of their breaking strength for 28 days after implantation and still retain 13 percent of their original strength at 56 days. In contrast, braided absorbable sutures retain only 1 to 5 percent of their strength at 28 days after implantation.[10]

SURGICAL NEEDLES

Surgical needles are produced from stainless steel alloys. A surgical needle has three basic components: the swage, body, and needle point (Fig. 10–1). The swage is the site of attachment of the suture. It provides a smooth juncture between the needle and suture, minimizing the size of the hole made in the tissue. The body of the needle is the portion that is grasped by the needle holder. The shape of the cross-sectional area and the configuration of its length categorize the needle body. The cross-sectional areas of the needle bodies may be circular, triangular, rectangular, or trapezoidal. The curvature of the needle is described in degrees of the subtended arc. The radius is the distance from the center of the circle to the body of the needle. The curvature of a needle with one radius of curvature may vary from 90 to 225 degrees. Needles with a curvature of 135 degrees are generally used to approximate the edges of traumatic lacerations. A 135-degree curvature (as shown in Fig. 10–1) enables a needle to pass through tissue with a limited rotation of the wrist. The 180-degree needle is ideally suited for use in deep body cavities, where a more limited arc of wrist rotation successfully passes the entire needle and provides sufficient exposure of the needle tip to allow for easy needle retrieval by the practitioner.

The point of the needle is at its tip. There are several types of needle tips: cutting edges, taper points, or a combination of both. Cutting-edge needles have two or more opposing edges and are designed to penetrate tough tissue. The position of a third cutting edge categorizes the needle as either a conventional cutting-edge needle or a reverse cutting-edge needle (Fig. 10–2). An inside cutting edge causes a linear cut that is perpendicular and close to the incision, against which the suture exerts a wound closure force that may ultimately cut through the tissue. In contrast, a reverse cutting edge cuts through

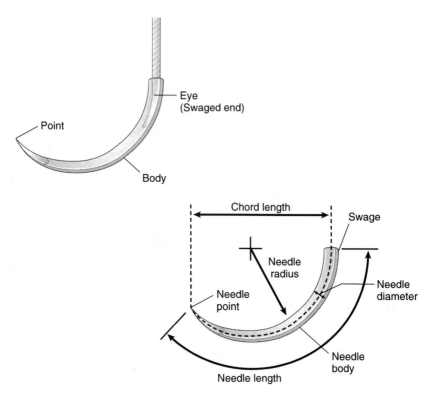

FIG. 10–1. *(Left)* Components and *(Right)* anatomy of a needle.

skin, leaving a wide wall of tissue (rather than an incision) against which the suture exerts its wound closure force. This wall of tissue resists suture cut-through.

The taper-point needle tapers to a sharp tip, which spreads the tissue without cutting it. Taper point needles are used in soft tissues that do not resist

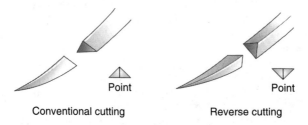

FIG. 10–2. A conventional cutting-edge surgical needle point has three cutting edges, with the apical cutting edge on the inside concave surface of the needle. A reverse cutting-edge needle point has three cutting edges, with the apical cutting edge on the outer convex surface.

needle penetration, such as vessels, abdominal viscera, and fascia. They are not generally used for repair of traumatic lacerations.

REFERENCES

1. Edlich, RF, Tsung, MS, Rogers, W, et al: Studies in management of the contaminated wound. I. Technique of closure of such wounds together with a note on a reproducible experimental model. J Surg Res 8:585–592, 1968.
2. Edlich, RF, Panek, PH, Rodeheaver, GT, et al: Physical and chemical configuration of sutures in the development of surgical infection. Ann Surg 177:679–688, 1973.
3. Sharp, WV, Belden, TA, King, PH, et al: Suture resistance to infection. Surgery 91:61–63, 1982.
4. Rodeheaver, GT, Borzelleca, DC, Thacker, JG, et al: Unique performance characteristics of Novafil. Surg Gynecol Obstet 164:230–236, 1987.
5. Pham, S, Rodeheaver, GT, Dang, MC, et al: Ease of continuous dermal suture removal. J Emerg Med 8:539–543, 1990.
6. Postlethwait, RW: Long-term comparative study of nonabsorbable sutures. Ann Surg 171:892–898, 1970.
7. Trimbos, JB, Smeets, M, Verdel, M, et al: Cosmetic result of lower midline laparotomy wounds: Polybutester and nylon in a randomized controlled trial. Obstet Gynecol 82:390–393, 1993.
8. Salthouse, TN, Williams, JA, and Willigan, DA: Relationship of cellular enzyme activity to catgut and collagen suture absorption. Surg Gynecol Obstet 29:691–696, 1969.
9. Rodeheaver, GT, Thacker, JG, and Edlich, RF: Mechanical performance of polyglycolic acid and polyglactin 910 synthetic absorbable sutures. Surg Gynecol Obstet 153:835–841, 1981.
10. Ray, JA, Doddi, N, Regula, D, et al: Polydioxanone (PDS), a novel monofilament synthetic absorbable suture. Surg Gynecol Obstet 153:497–507, 1981.
11. Rodeheaver, GT, Beltran KA, Green CW, et al: Biomechanical and clinical performance of a new synthetic monofilament absorbable suture. J Long Term Eff Med Implants 6:181–198, 1996.

ADAM J. SINGER, MD
LIOR ROSENBERG, MD

C H A P T E R

11

Basic Suturing and Tissue Handling Techniques

GENERAL PRINCIPLES

The ultimate goal of wound closure is to achieve a functional and cosmetically appealing scar. This is best achieved by gentle handling of all tissues to avoid further trauma, matching each layer of the wound with its corresponding counterpart on the opposite side, ensuring eversion of the wound edges, and minimizing the amount of tension on the wound. As the wound heals and the swelling subsides, the wound eventually flattens, becoming flush with the surrounding skin surface. Care should be taken to avoid an inverted or depressed scar, which will cast a shadow that will tend to accentuate the scar's width. Taking a larger bite at the depth of the wound than through the more superficial layers helps achieve wound eversion. Wound eversion is facilitated with the use of mattress or deep sutures. For most wounds, simple, interrupted percutaneous sutures, with or without interrupted dermal sutures, are all that is required.

TISSUE HANDLING

Increasing the amount of trauma to the wound edges and its surrounding skin increases the likelihood of infection and suboptimal cosmetic scar appearance.[1] Therefore, it is very important to avoid any further damage by carefully handling the traumatized tissues during repair. This can be achieved by minimizing the amount of tissue handling and using the least destructive surgical instruments. When available, skin hooks should be used instead of tissue forceps to help elevate and turn over the wound edges (Fig. 11-1). Care should be taken to avoid piercing the epidermis with the point of the skin hook. Excessive twisting or bending of the base of tissue flaps should also be avoided

108

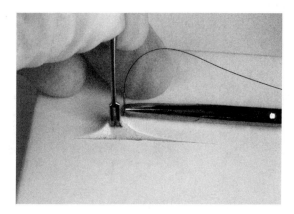

FIG. 11–1. A skin hook is used to elevate the wound edge, facilitating suture placement.

because it may reduce their blood flow. When skin hooks are not readily available, gentle forceps (e.g., Adson's forceps) with small teeth can be used to elevate the wound edges (Fig. 11–2). Whenever possible, the skin should be elevated using one arm of the forceps only. The wound edges should never be crushed between the forceps' arms and teeth. Alternatively, the skin can be grasped with the tissue forceps by its subcutaneous tissues, avoiding contact with the more superficial layers (see Fig. 11–2). Use of electrocautery should be minimized because it also increases the risk of infection and suboptimal appearance.[1] Hemostasis of the cutaneous vessels may be achieved

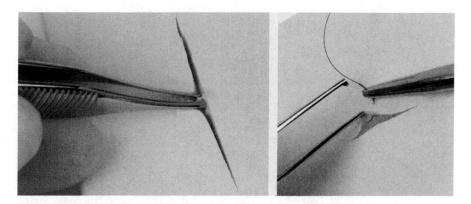

FIG. 11–2. *(Right)* While holding the tissue forceps in the non-dominant hand, the practitioner uses one arm of the tissue forceps to elevate the wound edge in the same manner as a skin hook. *(Left)* Alternatively, the subcutaneous tissue may be gently grasped.

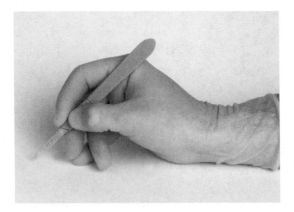

FIG. 11–3. A No. 15 blade is held like a pencil.

by gentle direct pressure, through the pressure produced by sutures, or by judicious use of bipolar electrocautery.

USE OF SCALPELS

The skin should always be cut using a sharp blade and smooth, continuous strokes. "Sawing" motions further traumatize the skin and should be avoided. The No. 15 blade is preferred for débridement of most small traumatic lacerations. It allows the most accurate incisions, particularly those that are angular or irregular. The blade should enter the skin at a 90-degree angle. Its handle should be held like a pencil between the thumb and index finger supported by the middle finger of the dominant hand (Fig. 11–3). The No. 10 blade is rarely used in the acute setting. Its rounded belly edge is mainly used to perform long, linear incisions in the operating room. The No. 10 scalpel is classically held like a violin's bowstring (Fig. 11–4), but it can also be held like a pencil for more accurate incisions.

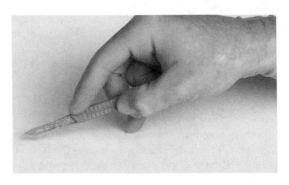

FIG. 11–4. A No. 10 blade is held like the bowstring of a violin.

BASIC SUTURING TECHNIQUES

Generally, the preferred method for tying sutures when closing the skin is the instrument tie using a needle holder. Instrument ties are more rapid and accurate than hand ties and can be used in recesses that do not allow hand tying. The major disadvantage to tying with instruments is the inability to apply continuous tension to the suture ends. As a result, there may be slippage of the suture knots with loosening of the closure in wounds subject to tension. In principle, the wound should never be closed under tension. Using intradermal sutures at different layers helps distribute the tension over a greater number of sutures. **To avoid slippage of the suture, the first knot should be constructed using a double throw.** Hand tying should be considered when using large sutures (i.e., larger than 2-0) and when done by those who have not mastered the instrument tie. Hand ties should be used only rarely in wounds subject to very large static tensions.

CHOOSING A NEEDLE HOLDER

Straight surgical needles are almost never used in the acute setting. The curved surgical needles that are used require the use of a needle holder. Many needle holders have small teeth along their jaws to prevent the needle from slipping.[2] However, these teeth can damage or tear the suture material.[3] Using needle holders with smooth jaws eliminates these problems, but the needle may slip.[4] A good option (when they are available) is specialized needle holders in which the texture of their jaws has been altered.[5]

HOLDING A NEEDLE HOLDER

The needle holder may be held by one of two methods. In the thumb–ring finger grip, the ring finger is inserted in the lower ringlet of the needle holder and serves as the pivot point around which the instrument rotates. The tip of the thumb's distal volar pad is positioned on the inner side of the upper ringlet, stabilizing it and facilitating the release of the ratchet mechanism (Fig. 11–5). This grip allows controlled movement of the needle holder and an accurate and controlled disengagement of the ratchet mechanism when releasing the needle. This precise needle manipulation and avoidance of inadvertent motion during the release process is crucial for the accurate placement of sutures. This grip, in which the hand is separated from the needle holder, may be a little difficult to master at first, but it is worth learning because of its precision.

In the thenar grip, the needle holder is grasped in the palm of the hand without inserting the tips of the thumb and ring fingers into the needle holder ringlets (Fig. 11–6). In this position, the needle holder is held in the palm between the thenar eminence and the second to fifth fingers. The major advantage of this grip is its versatility, allowing the needle holder to be comfortably positioned in difficult areas such as recessed cavities. Its major disadvantage is the loss of precision when the thenar eminence applies pressure to the ringlet to disengage the ratchet mechanism. This pressure may cause slight

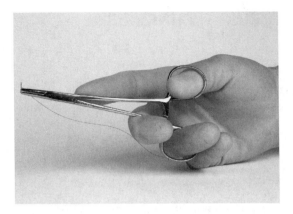

FIG. 11–5. The thumb–ring finger grip for a needle holder.

movement of the needle. The thenar grip should only be used after mastering the thumb–ring finger grip.

The needle should be pushed through the tissues following the direction of its curvature. Pushing the needle in a different vector than its curvature will result in "plowing" of the tissue and further trauma. This "plowing" motion may also bend or break the needle.

SIMPLE INTERRUPTED PERCUTANEOUS SUTURES AND INSTRUMENT TIES

The advantages and disadvantages of the various suturing methods are summarized in Table 11–1. **The simple interrupted suture is the most commonly**

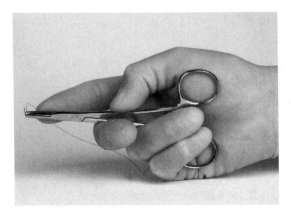

FIG. 11–6. The thenar grip for a needle holder.

TABLE 11–1. ADVANTAGES AND DISADVANTAGES OF VARIOUS SUTURING METHODS			
Suture Type	**Advantages**	**Disadvantages**	**Frequent Uses**
Interrupted percutaneous	Excellent approximation	Time consuming May strangulate tissues	Low-tension wounds May be used with deep sutures for high-tension wounds
Continuous percutaneous	Rapid closure Accommodates edema	Less meticulous closure than interrupted sutures If a single knot unravels, the wound may dehisce (if no deep sutures are placed)	Percutaneous closure in conjunction with deep sutures
Interrupted dermal	Reduces tension on wound surface Allows early removal of percutaneous sutures, avoiding hatchmarking May reduce scar width	May increase infection in contaminated wounds	High-tension wounds Closure of dead space
Continuous dermal	Rapid Reduces tension on wound surface Allows early removal of percutaneous sutures, avoiding hatchmarking May reduce scar width	Technically difficult Less accurate approximation than interrupted sutures If a single knot unravels, the wound may dehisce	High-tension wounds require interrupted dermal sutures Closure of dead space

(continues)

TABLE 11–1. ADVANTAGES AND DISADVANTAGES OF VARIOUS SUTURING METHODS (Continued)

Suture Type	Advantages	Disadvantages	Frequent Uses
Vertical mattress	Excellent wound edge eversion Combines advantages of deep and superficial sutures	May cause tissue strangulation	Thin or lax skin with little dermal or fascial tissue High-tension areas (e.g., extremities)
Horizontal mattress	More rapid than simple interrupted sutures Excellent wound edge eversion	May cause tissue strangulation	Bleeding scalp wounds Initial approximation of high-tension wounds
Half-buried, horizontal mattress	Less compromising to flap perfusion	Time consuming Technically difficult	Corner stitches and flaps

used method of closing cutaneous wounds.[6] In one series[7] of more than 5000 traumatic lacerations (before the introduction of tissue adhesives), 78 percent were repaired by simple interrupted sutures, 8 percent using staples, 4 percent using vertical mattress sutures, 3 percent using adhesive tapes, 2 percent using running sutures, and 1 percent using horizontal mattress sutures. **The simple interrupted suture is most appropriate for closing the outer layers of the skin when the laceration or incision is under minimal tension.** It also results in the most meticulous apposition of the edges of the wound.

The needle is grasped with the tip of the needle holder approximately one half to one third of the distance from the attachment of the suture to the needle and the needle's tip, and the ratchet mechanism is engaged with one click (Fig. 11–7). To insert simple interrupted sutures, the needle should be passed so that more tissue is included at the depth of the wound than at the surface, resulting in a pear-shaped loop when the wound is viewed in cross-section (Fig. 11–8). This procedure promotes eversion of the skin edges. It is best achieved by entering the skin at an angle of 90 degrees (see Fig. 11–7) and is facilitated by starting with the hand in full pronation and supinating the wrist during the passage of the needle through the skin.

Eversion of the skin edges is thought to avoid a depressed scar by opposing the tendency of the approximated wound edges to contract downward during healing. For right-handed practitioners, the needle should usually enter the right or far side of the wound and exit through the middle of the wound. The needle is than grasped with the tip of the needle holder and

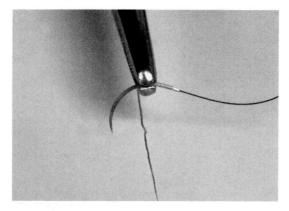

FIG. 11–7. The needle is held by the jaws of the needle holder approximately one-third to one-half of the distance from the junction of the suture and needle. The needle enters the skin at a 90-degree angle.

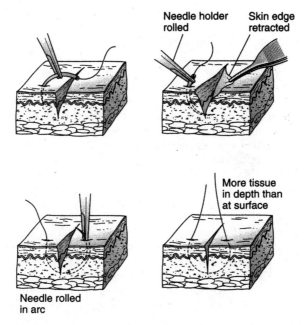

FIG. 11–8. Cross section of wound demonstrating proper suture placement. The distance of the suture from the wound edge is greater at the depth of the wound than near its surface. (From Singer AS, Burstein JL, and Schiavone FM: Emergency Medicine Pearls, ed 2. Philadelphia, F.A. Davis, 2001, p 208, with permission.)

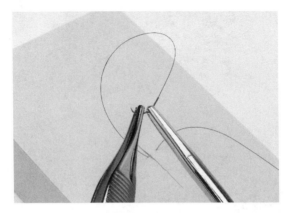

FIG. 11–9. The needle is grasped by the forceps and rearmed within the jaws of the needle holder.

rearmed using a tissue forceps (Fig. 11–9). When not in use, the tissue forceps may be held in the palm of the nondominant hand to maximize the practitioner's efficiency. The needle is then passed through the other side of the wound, starting at its depth and exiting through the skin's surface. The needle should enter and exit the skin at exactly the same levels and distances on either side of the wound in order to achieve accurate approximation and matching of the various levels of the skin. When the wound edges are uneven, with one being less stable than the other (e.g., with a flap), the needle should first be passed through the less stable side. If this is on the left or near side of the wound, the practitioner should use a backhanded approach in which the wrist is fully supinated and the needle is passed by pronating the wrist (Fig. 11–10A). Note that with this approach, the needle should be loaded with its tip pointing to the right side of the needle holder (Fig. 11–10B).

After exiting the second side of the wound, the suture should be advanced through the tissue until only its distal 2 to 4 cm remains within the skin. This makes it easier to form a loop. To avoid getting entangled when the suture is still very long, the practitioner may drop the needle with the loose suture on the surgical field and grasp the suture material approximately 10 to 20 cm away from the wound (Fig. 11–11).

When tying the first knot, the fixed end of the suture should be wrapped twice around the tip of the needle holder in a clockwise direction with the nondominant hand (Fig. 11–12). The free end of the suture should then be grasped with the jaws of the needle holder, and the ratchet mechanism should be engaged. The tip of the suture should then be pulled through the suture loop across the wound while the fixed end is also pulled across the wound in the opposite direction (Fig. 11–13). The suture loop may be tightened by pulling on the suture ends so the knot does not slip. When there is no tension on the wound edges and the placement of the suture is relatively easy, one may tie the first knot as a double knot and lock it with an oppositely directed single knot. This creates a flat "surgeon's knot," which prevents slippage of the first throw when tension is applied to the wound edges.

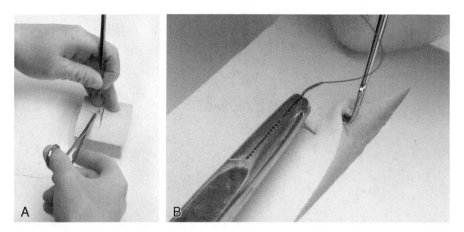

FIG. 11–10. (A) Backhand approach to inserting needle from the left or near side of the wound. (B) Note that the needle is armed with its tip pointing to the right of the needle holder.

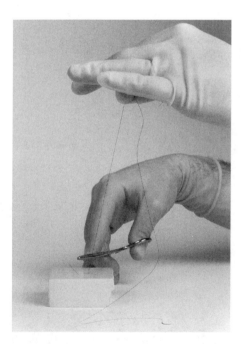

FIG. 11–11. The suture material may be grasped at its center to avoid getting entangled when very long.

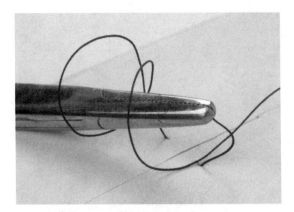

FIG. 11–12. The first throw is formed by looping the fixed end of the suture twice around the tip of the needle holder in a clockwise direction.

The second tie is created in reverse by looping the fixed end of the suture once around the tip of the needle holder in a counterclockwise direction (Fig. 11–14). The tip of the suture is then grasped with the needle holder and the tip is pulled through the second suture loop across the wound while the other end of the suture is pulled across the wound in the opposite direction (Fig. 11–15). This creates a flat knot. Additional ties are placed alternating the direction in which the suture is wrapped around the needle holder, and the hands are crossed when pulling the suture across the wounds, creating multiple square, flat knots. **Generally, the number of ties should correspond with the suture size.** For example, with unbraided nylon, use no fewer than five ties for a 5-0 suture, six ties for a 6-0 suture, and so forth. The knots should

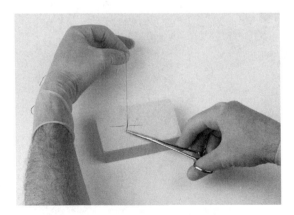

FIG. 11–13. The tip of the suture is grasped with the needle holder and pulled across the wound. Note that the nondominant hand is pulling the fixed end of the suture in the opposite direction, creating a flat knot.

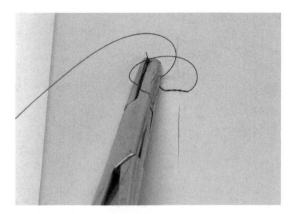

FIG. 11–14. The second tie is formed by looping the fixed end around the free end in a counterclockwise direction.

be tied tightly enough to appose the wound edges, yet not so tight that they strangulate the tissues.[8] The ends of the suture should be cut leaving an ear that is shorter than the distance between sutures (usually 3 to 5 mm long) to facilitate removal and avoid getting them entangled with each other.

The first suture should be placed at the center of the wound. Additional sutures are then placed midway between the center of the wound and its corners. This process of bisecting the remaining limbs of the wound with sutures is continued until apposition of the wound edges is achieved (Fig. 11–16). Because the presence of suture material increases the likelihood of infection,[9] the number of sutures should be kept at a minimum.

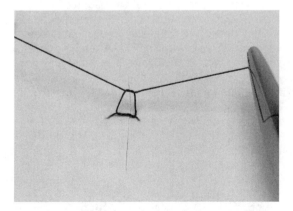

FIG. 11–15. After forming the second tie, the two hands should move in opposite directions, pulling the suture across the wound and creating a flat knot.

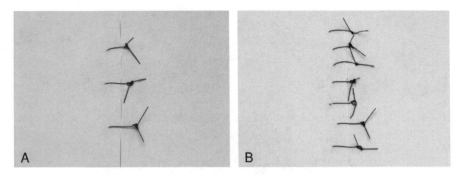

FIG. 11–16. (*A* and *B*) The first suture is placed at the center of the wound. The remaining limbs are sequentially bisected with additional sutures till wound apposition is complete.

SIMPLE INTERRUPTED DERMAL SUTURES

Simple interrupted dermal sutures are used to close the dermis. They are placed in wounds that are subject to large static tensions to reduce the tendency for these wounds to form wide scars or to dehisce. **Using dermal sutures also allows early removal of the percutaneous sutures before the formation of ugly suture marks.** Deep sutures should be used judiciously, however, because they have been shown to increase infection rates in contaminated wounds.[10] For most deep sutures, an absorbable suture that remains within the wound for at least 4 to 6 weeks is required (see Chapter 10).

   Deep sutures should be placed so that the knot is buried at the depth of the wound. This is accomplished by starting and ending suture placement at the depth of the wound. The deep suture is placed by entering the wound at the reticular dermis and exiting beneath the dermal–epidermal junction on the left or near side of the wound (Fig. 11–17). After exiting the first side of the wound and rearming the needle holder, the needle is then inserted on the other side of the wound immediately beneath the epidermal–dermal junction and exits at the lower portion of the reticular dermis at exactly the same level on the contralateral side (see Fig. 11–17). After placing the suture, a knot should be formed using four or five throws. When tying the knot, the hands should move in a direction parallel to the wound (Fig. 11–18). **The deep suture should then be cut as close to the knot as possible.** To avoid premature unraveling of the suture caused by very short tail ends, one additional throw should be added before cutting the suture.[11] With long wounds, several dermal sutures may be required. The first suture should be placed at the center of the wound, with sequential bisection of the remaining limbs of the wound as described earlier.

CONTINUOUS PERCUTANEOUS SUTURES

With continuous sutures, the entire wound is closed before dividing the suture material. The major advantages of continuous sutures are their relative speed

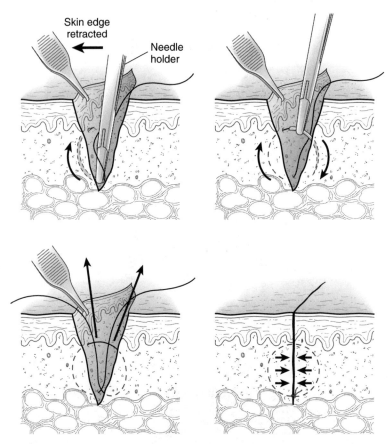

FIG. 11–17. Placement of a deep suture. The needle is inserted at the depth of the dermis and directed upward, exiting immediately beneath the dermal-epidermal junction. The needle is then inserted through the opposite side of the wound, starting at the dermal-epidermal junction and exiting at the depth of the dermis.

and the ability to adapt to progressive swelling of the wound. They are particularly useful for long linear wounds. It is difficult to control the distribution of tension along the wound, however. It is also difficult to achieve perfect apposition of the wound edges, so continuous sutures should not be used for irregular wounds and should not be used by novices. This type of suture does not play a major role in the acute setting.

The first suture, similar to a simple interrupted percutaneous suture, is placed at one end of the wound. After completing the first knot, the suture material is not divided. The needle is then inserted next to the first suture at the opposite side of the wound, crossing the wound at a 65-degree angle (Fig. 11–19). The needle then crosses the depth of the wound in a circular motion perpendicular to the wound, exiting on the opposite side approximately 3 to 5 mm from the wound edge. This process is repeated as needed until the entire wound is approximated. After placing the last suture, a small loop is left,

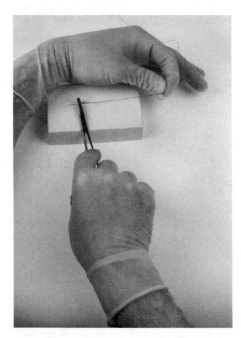

FIG. 11–18. Tying the knot of a deep suture. The hands move in a direction parallel to the wound.

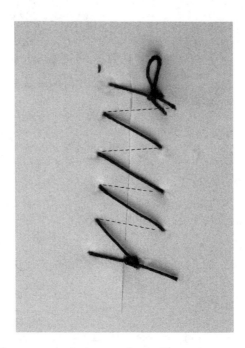

FIG. 11–19. Continuous percutaneous sutures. The suture crosses the wound superficially at a 65-degree angle. The suture traverses the depth of the wound at a 90-degree angle.

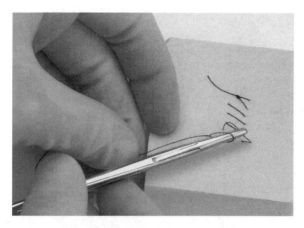

FIG. 11–20. After completing placement of the continuous percutaneous suture, the knot is formed by grasping a loop of suture.

which serves as an anchor for tying the knot (Fig. 11–20). The knot itself is constructed as previously described. To ensure knot security, at least five or six throws should be used.[12]

CONTINUOUS DERMAL SUTURES

Continuous dermal sutures are the most technically complex sutures. When the technique is mastered, they allow excellent wound closure and excellent cosmesis without the need for percutaneous sutures. This is particularly advantageous for frightened children, patients in whom suture removal is problematic, and patients with a tendency to form hypertrophic scars or keloids. They are also very useful when the wound will be under a cast or splint, precluding their early removal. Continuous dermal sutures are also appropriate for wounds subject to large dynamic or static tensions. Obviously, there is no risk for suture marks using this method of closure. They have not been shown to reduce scar width, however,[13] and their use may be associated with higher wound infection rates.[14] **An alternative to continuous dermal sutures is a combination of interrupted dermal sutures and tissue adhesives.**

Before placing a continuous dermal suture, it is helpful to place several deep dermal sutures along the wound to reduce tension and align the wound edges in an optimal position, every 2 to 5 cm. One tail of these interrupted dermal sutures should be left longer for anchoring of the continuous dermal suture (Fig. 11–21). A deep suture is also placed at the corner of the wound to anchor the last continuous suture. When constructing a continuous dermal suture, the suture should first be anchored in the skin by entering the subcutaneous tissue at one end of the wound (usually on the right or farthest side in the case of a right-handed practitioner) and exiting in the lower dermis (Fig. 11–22). A five-throw knot is tied, and the end is cut. The needle is then inserted below the epidermal–dermal junction on one side of the wound and passed in

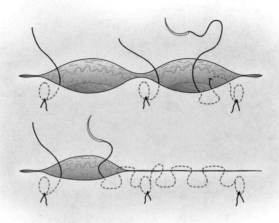

FIG. 11–21. Placement of interrupted dermal sutures prior to a continuous dermal suture (*upper*). A long tail is left with each suture as an anchor for the more superficial continuous intradermal suture (*lower*).

a horizontal direction parallel to the wound surface (Fig. 11–23). After exiting the upper dermis, the needle is backtracked 1 or 2 mm and inserted on the other side of the wound through the upper dermis in a horizontal direction as before.

This process is repeated using small bites, passing above the interrupted dermal sutures, intermittently tying the suture to the long tail ends of the dermal sutures that were placed for this purpose (see Fig. 11–21) until the wound is closed. Careful yet steady traction on the fixed end of the suture while pro-

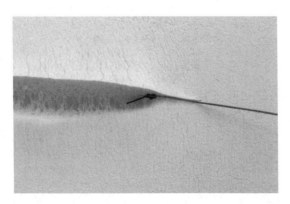

FIG. 11–22. Placement of a continuous dermal suture. The suture is anchored at the apex of the wound.

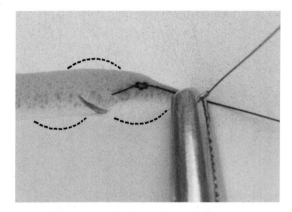

FIG. 11–23. Placement of the continuous dermal suture. Small horizontal bites are taken beneath the dermal-epidermal junction. Slight backtracking of the needle path should be performed to ensure wound coaptation.

gressing helps to approximate the wound edges. When the last suture is passed, it is tied to the long tail of the last interrupted dermal suture (see Fig. 11–21). With short or tension-free wounds, the practitioner may choose to place continuous dermal sutures without underlying interrupted dermal sutures. In this case, the last suture is tied using a small loop of the suture to anchor the knot, similar to a continuous percutaneous suture (Fig. 11–24). After tying the knot, the suture is cut and buried beneath the skin by passing the needle and fixed end of the suture through the wound, exiting through the skin at a distance from the end of the wound (Fig. 11–25). After applying tension on the fixed end of the suture, the suture is cut flush with the skin, and its end retracts beneath the surface.

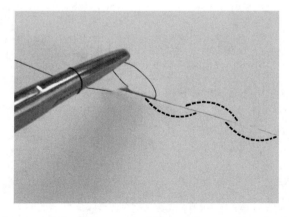

FIG. 11–24. After completing placement of the continuous dermal suture, the knot is tied by grasping a loop of suture material.

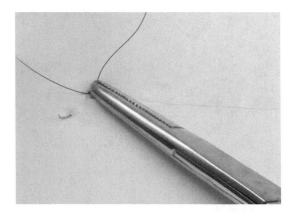

FIG. 11–25. The knot is buried in the subcutaneous tissue by inserting the needle at the wound depth and exiting approximately 5 mm from the wound edge.

SPECIAL SUTURES AND SITUATIONS

MATTRESS SUTURES

When approximation and eversion of the wound's edges is difficult, interrupted or continuous mattress sutures may also be used to close the skin. With *vertical mattress* sutures, the first bite is a large one, which includes equal amounts of tissue from either side of the wound, extending 1 cm outward from each side. The needle is then reversed, and a smaller, more superficial backhanded bite is taken 1 to 2 mm from the wound edges (Fig. 11–26). Alternatively, vertical mattress sutures may be placed by starting with the small bite. After elevating the wound edges by traction on the first suture ends, a second, deep bite is taken.[15] This method is more rapid than the first, but the second bite is passed blindly, risking injury to underlying structures.

Vertical mattress sutures serve two functions: (1) the large bite results in a secure grasp of tissue, and (2) the small bite achieves meticulous approximation of the skin edges. This suture results in excellent wound edge eversion. Vertical mattress sutures are particularly useful in very thin or lax skin and in areas (e.g., over the shins) where the deep subcutaneous tissues are too poor to be used for anchoring tension-reducing sutures. **Vertical mattress sutures also may be indicated when the wound edges tend to invert on closure.** One of the major disadvantages of vertical mattress sutures, however, is that they may result in too much tension on the more superficial skin edges, which reduces blood supply to the skin. The ischemic skin may then undergo necrosis and become macerated, inviting infection, interfering with the healing process, and resulting in a poor scar.

With a *horizontal mattress* suture, the first bite is placed similar to a simple interrupted suture. Before tying a knot, however, a second bite is taken adjacent to the first one by reversing the direction of the needle (Fig. 11–27). This suture also results in wound edge eversion, but the skin that is caught within each horizontal bite may lose its circulation, resulting in necrosis. However, initial placement of a horizontal mattress suture in the middle of the wound before closure

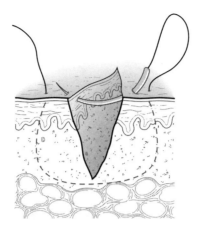

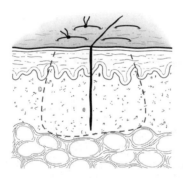

FIG. 11–26. Formation of a vertical mattress suture. The first bite is taken far from the wound. The direction of the needle is reversed and a second bite is taken close to the wound edge. (From Singer AS, Burstein JL, and Schiavone FM: Emergency Medicine Pearls, ed 2. Philadelphia, F.A. Davis, 2001, p 209, with permission.)

with simple interrupted sutures makes it easier to obtain wound edge eversion. **Horizontal mattress sutures can be used by novice practicioners as temporary sutures to facilitate wound edge eversion before initiating repair with simple sutures.** After placement of the simple sutures, the initial horizontal mattress suture can be removed and replaced with two simple interrupted sutures. This method facilitates excellent eversion that sometimes cannot be accomplished with simple sutures alone. The two horizontal and vertical mattress sutures may also be combined into an oblique mattress suture.

CLOSING WOUNDS WITH EDGES OF UNEVEN LENGTHS

When the lengths of the two opposite sides of a wound are uneven, simple closure may result in distortion of adjacent skin, resulting in formation of a "dog

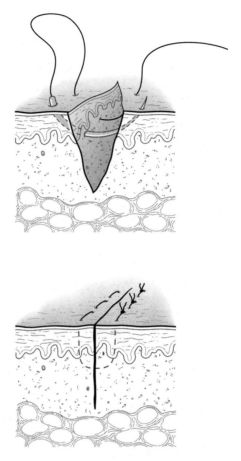

FIG. 11–27. Formation of a horizontal mattress suture. The first bite is taken and the needle is reversed and a second bite is taken.

ear." This may be avoided by placing the first suture in the exact midpoint of *each side* of the wound. Before tying the knot, it is helpful to hold the wound edges together with the suture that was placed in the middle of the wound to see if the edges are properly aligned. If the positioning is satisfactory, the knot is tied and the remaining sutures are placed by sequentially placing bisecting sutures in the remaining halves of the wound.

Another method to close wounds with uneven lengths without ending up with a dog ear is to place the sutures farther apart on the longer side of the wound (Fig. 11–28). However, sometimes a dog ear is unavoidable. One method for managing a dog ear is presented in Fig. 11–29; however, this method does elongate the scar.

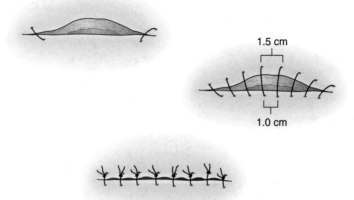

FIG. 11–28. Alternative method for closing wounds whose edges are of uneven lengths. The distances between sutures on the longer side are greater than on the shorter side.

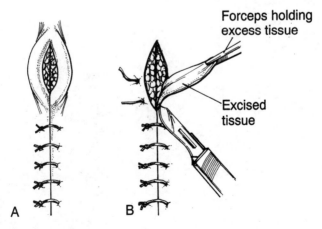

FIG. 11–29. Method for managing a dog ear. The excessive tissue is removed with an elliptical incision and the resulting wound is closed. (From Singer AS, Burstein JL, and Schiavone FM: Emergency Medicine Pearls, ed 2. Philadelphia, F.A. Davis, 2001, p 209, with permission.)

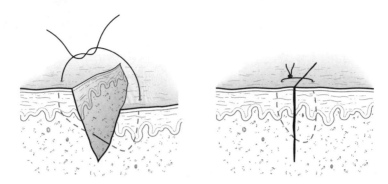

FIG. 11–30. Closing wounds with surfaces on different levels. A "deeper" bite is taken from the depressed side, elevating it.

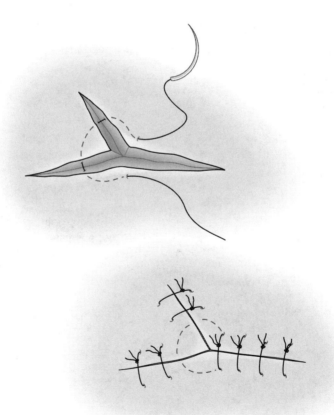

FIG. 11–31. The half-buried horizontal mattress suture for closing corners and flaps. The needle is passed underneath the epidermis at the tip of the flap. The needle should enter and exit at the same level of the dermis on either side of the wound.

CLOSING WOUNDS WITH SURFACES THAT ARE NOT LEVEL

When one side of the wound is elevated and the other is depressed, deeper "bites" should be taken from the depressed side of the wound by inserting the needle at a deeper level on the depressed side (Fig. 11–30). This elevates that side.

CORNER STITCHES AND CLOSURE OF FLAPS

At times, the wound creates a flap or multiple flaps with narrow, poorly vascularized bases. This may occur, for example, with lacerations in the shape of a "V," "Y," or "X." Placement of percutaneous sutures through the end of such flaps may further compromise blood flow and cause necrosis of the skin at the tip. This outcome can be avoided by placing a half-buried, circular horizontal mattress suture in which the suture material is placed in the subcuticular region of the flap (Fig. 11–31).

UNDERMINING

Occasionally, high tension on the wound makes it difficult to approximate wound edges. The amount of tension on the wound may be reduced by undermining the areas of the skin on either side of the wound. With undermining, tissue is recruited by cutting the attachment of the dermis and superficial

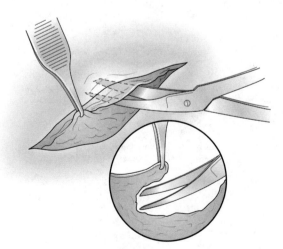

FIG. 11–32. Method of tissue undermining. The superficial skin is released from the deeper subcutaneous structure with scissors or by sweeping a No. 15 blade below the dermis.

fascia from deeper structures, which then allows a tension-free closure. The dissection should occur in the subdermal plane below the subdermal plexus (Fig. 11–32). An upward scraping motion on the undersurface of the dermis is helpful when using a blade.

Undermining may be performed with scissors (either iris or Metzenbaum scissors) or with a No. 15 scalpel. For accurate dissection, the skin to be undermined must be pulled forward following the direction of the skin, not flipped backward to expose the deeper tissues. The skin should be pulled forward with a skin hook rather than with forceps. If no skin hook is available, one can be fashioned by using forceps to bend back the point of a 21-gauge needle.

REFERENCES

1. Singer, AJ, Quinn, JV, Clark, RE, et al: Determinants of poor outcome after laceration and incision repair. Plast Reconstr Surg, 2002 (in press).
2. Thacker, JG, Borzelleca, DC, Hunter, JC, et al: Biomechanical analysis of needle holding security. J Biomed Mater Res 20:903–917, 1986.
3. Stamp, CV, McGregor, W, Rodeheaver, GT, et al: Surgical needle holder damage to sutures. Am Surg 54:300–306, 1988.
4. Bond, RF, McGregor, W, Cutler, PV, et al: Influence of needle holder jaw configuration on the biomechanics of curved surgical needle bending. J Appl Biomater 1:39–47, 1990.
5. Abidin, MR, Dunlapp, JA, Towler, MA, et al: Metallurgically bonded needle holder jaws: A technique to enhance needle holding security without sutural damage. Am Surg 56:643–657, 1990.
6. Hollander, JE, Singer, AJ, Valentine, S, et al: Wound registry: Development and validation. Ann Emerg Med 25:675–685, 1995.
7. Hollander, JE, Valentine, S, Singer, and AJ: Characteristics of traumatic lacerations and their influence on post-repair infection rate (abstract). Acad Emerg Med 5:466, 1998.
8. Myers, BM, and Cherry, G: Functional and angiographic vasculature in healing wounds. Am Surg 36:750–756, 1970.
9. Edlich, RF, Panek, PH, Rodeheaver, GT, et al: Physical and chemical configuration of sutures in the development of surgical infection. Ann Surg 177:679–688, 1973.
10. Mehta, PH, Dunn, KA, Bradfield, JF, et al: Contaminated wounds: infection rates with subcutaneous sutures. Ann Emerg Med 27:43–48, 1996.
11. Mazzarese, PM, Faulkner, BC, Gear, AJL, et al: Technical considerations in knot construction. Part II. Interrupted dermal suture closure. J Emerg Med 15:505–511, 1999.
12. Annunziata, CC, Drake, DB, Woods, JA, et al: Technical considerations in knot construction. Part I. Continuous percutaneous and dermal suture closure. J Emerg Med 15:351–356, 1999.
13. Winn, HR, Jane, RA, Rodeheaver, H, et al: Influence of subcuticular sutures on scar formation. Am J Surg 133:257–259, 1977.
14. Foster, GE, Hardy, EG, and Hardcastle, JD: Subcuticular suturing after appendectomy. Lancet 1:1128–1129, 1977.
15. Jones, JS, Gartner, M, Drew, G, et al: The shorthand vertical mattress stitch: Evaluation of a new suture technique. Am J Emerg Med 11:483–485, 1993.

DANIEL J. DIRE, MD, FACEP

C H A P T E R

12

Animal Bites

Handwritten notes:
Dog bite : pasteurella
Cat bite : pasteurella
cat scratch : bartonella
human bite : Staph, strep
Eikenella

Every year, an estimated 1 to 2 million animal bites are treated in the United States, including 10 to 20 deaths from dog attacks. A survey of emergency departments reported that there were 333,687 injuries related to dog bites treated annually.[1] The goals in treating these wounds are to restore function, provide good cosmetic results, and prevent infection.

The true incidence of animal bites may never be known. Not all bite victims seek medical care, many because of the trivial nature of their wounds. This may be true especially for those who have been bitten by cats or other small animals because these wounds are more often small puncture wounds that do not prompt the victim to be concerned.

The most frequent complication from bites is infection. Infection rates of 1.4 to 30 percent have been reported from dog bites,[2-6] 15.6 to 50 percent from cat bites,[7,8] and 9 to 18 percent from human bites.[9-11] Other diseases transmitted by animal bites include cat scratch fever (*Bartonella henselae*), tularemia (*Francisella tularensis*), leptospirosis, brucellosis, and rat bite fever (*Spirillum minus*). Human bites can transmit hepatitis B, hepatitis C, syphilis, herpes simplex, tuberculosis, actinomycosis, tetanus, and human immunodeficiency virus (HIV) infections.

DOG BITES

Dog bites account for 63 to 93 percent of reported animal bites in humans.[6,12] Dog bite victims tend most often to be young boys and young men.[6,13] Pediatric dog bite victims acquire mostly head, neck, and upper extremity wounds, but adults who are bitten have mostly upper and lower extremity injuries with a low incidence of facial wounds.[6,14] Dogs have large teeth that crush and tear tissue. In patients with dog bite injuries, lacerations are seen in 31 to 45 percent, puncture wounds in 13 to 34 percent, and superficial abrasions in 30 to 43 percent.[6,15,16] Wound closure is required in 12 percent of patients.[6]

Dog bites are provoked in 33 to 94 percent of dog injuries.[6] Dogs exhibit territorial behavior, and victims may unknowingly provoke the attacks. Children often become victims when they approach, disturb, or play recklessly around resting or feeding animals or when they tease or attempt to kiss the animals.

BACTERIOLOGY

The bacteriology of dog bite wounds is complex. Wound infections do not usually result from the normal bacterial flora found on the patient's skin; rather, they usually result from the organisms inoculated into the depth of the wound by the dog's teeth. Aerobic bacteria have been isolated from 74 percent of fresh dog bite wounds, and anaerobic bacteria have been isolated from 41 percent.[3,17] *Staphylococcus aureus* is found in 72 percent of cultured nasal and oral secretions of dogs, and *Pasteurella multocida* is found in 66 percent.[18] A total of 66 percent of canine gingival scrapings reveal *Pasteurella* spp. (*P. stomatisis* in 68 percent, P. *multocida* in percent, P. *dagmatis* in 11 percent, and P. *canis* in 7 percent).[19]

Pasteurella spp. are the pathogens most frequently isolated from infected wounds (50 percent to 53 percent).[6,20] *Streptococcus* spp. are found in 29 percent, and *Staphylococcus aureus* is found in 20 to 29 percent. **Cultures of initially uninfected bite wounds are of no benefit in predicting the results of subsequent cultures of infected wounds.** Organisms recovered from dog bite wounds are listed in Table 12–1. The bacteriology of dog bite wound infections is frequently polymicrobial, and the types of infecting organisms vary from one geographic region to another.

Pasteurella multocida is a small, nonmotile, gram-negative coccobacillus that is of low virulence in humans. It acts as an opportunistic pathogen. Wound infections caused by these organisms are characterized by a rapidly developing, intense inflammatory response, which usually becomes symptomatic within 24 hours of injury. Pain and edema are prominent, but purulent drainage occurs in only 40 percent, lymphangitis in about 20 percent, and regional adenopathy in 10 percent of patients.[21] Septic arthritis is common when a canine tooth penetrates a joint, especially in the hand. Osteomyelitis, sepsis, meningitis, and abscess formation may complicate animal bites caused by this organism. The development of bacteremia after a patient is bitten is usually associated with immunocompromised states such as liver dysfunction and malignancy. Septicemia, pneumonia, and peritonitis have occurred after bites in patients with AIDS. *Pasteurella* spp. is most sensitive to penicillin G and its derivatives, second- and third- generation cephalosporins, tetracyclines, chloramphenicol, fluoroquinolones (ciprofloxacin, ofloxacin, enoxacin, levofloxacin), trimethoprim-sulfamethoxazole, clarithromycin, and azithromycin.[22,23] It is less susceptible to first-generation cephalosporins, semisynthetic penicillins, and erythromycin.

Capnocytophaga canimorsus is a fastidious, gram-negative bacillus found in the normal oral flora of dogs. C. *canimorsus* sepsis with disseminated intravascular coagulopathy, renal and multiorgan failure, and cutaneous gangrene has been reported in patients with asplenia, liver disease, or immunosuppression, as

TABLE 12–1. ORGANISMS RECOVERED FROM DOG AND CAT BITE WOUNDS

Dog Bites	Cat Bites

Aerobic Organisms

Dog Bites	Cat Bites
Aeromonas hydrophila	*Acinetobacter* spp.
Acinetobacter spp.	*Aeromonas hydrophila*
Actinobacillus spp.	*Alcaligenes faecalis*
Alpha Streptococcus	*Alcaligenes odorans*
Bacillis spp.	*Corynebacterium* spp.
Beta Streptococcus	*Enterobacter cloacae*
Blastomyces dermatitis	*Erysipelothrix rhusiopathiae*
Brucella canis	*Neisseria* spp.
Capnocytophaga canimorsus	*Pasteurella multocida* and other spp.
CDC alphanumeric groups:	*Panteoa agglomerans*
EF-4, IIj, IIr, M-5	*Rhodococcus* spp.
Chromobacterium spp.	*Staphylococcus aureus*
Corynebacterium spp.	*Staphylococcus epidermidis*
Escherichia coli	and other spp.
Enterobacter cloacae	*Streptococcus* spp.
Enterococcus spp.	*Streptomyces* spp.
Gamma Streptococcus	*Reimerella anatipestifer*
Haemophilus aphrophilus	*Tothia dentocariosa*
Klebsiella spp.	
Micrococcus luteus	
Moraxella spp.	
Neisseria spp.	
Pasteurella multocida and other spp.	
Proteus mirabilis	
Pseudomonas spp.	
Staphylococcus aureus, epidermidis,	
and *intermedius*	

Anaerobic Organisms

Dog Bites	Cat Bites
Bacteroides spp.	*Bacteroides* spp.
Eubacterium spp.	*Clostridium sordelli*
Fusobacterium spp.	*Filifactor villosus*
Lactobacillus jensenii	*Fusobacterium nucleatum*
Leptotrichia bacillus	*Peptostreptococcus* spp.
Peptococcus spp.	*Porphyromonas* spp.
Peptostreptococcus spp.	*Prevotella* spp.
Porphyromonas spp.	*Propionibacterium* spp.
Prevotella spp.	*Veillonella* spp.
Propionibacterium spp.	
Veillonella parvula	

well as in healthy hosts. The fatality rate is 25 percent. The antibiotic of choice is penicillin G, but the organism is also susceptible to ampicillin, carbenicillin, cephalothin, cefoxitin, cefotaxime, clindamycin, erythromycin, tetracycline, chloramphenicol, and ciprofloxacin.

TREATMENT

After appropriate wound preparation, uncomplicated bite lacerations of the head and neck can undergo primary repair without the use of prophylactic antibiotics. Contaminated bite wounds and puncture wounds should not be closed. The role of antibiotic agents in the treatment of patients who present with uninfected dog bites is controversial because of a paucity of published, prospective clinical data that address the issues of antibiotic choices, route of administration, and duration of therapy. A meta-analysis[24] of eight randomized trials of antibiotic agents to prevent infection in patients with dog bite wounds showed that the relative risk for infection was 0.58. Callaham[25] subsequently analyzed these data and concluded that it is not cost effective to prescribe prophylactic antibiotic agents for all patients who present without infection. **Antibiotics should not be prescribed as a substitute for meticulous wound cleansing and débridement.**

It is recommended that a prophylactic antibiotic agent be given to dog-bite victims with special conditions listed in Table 12–2 and in patients with higher-risk wounds. Until definitive studies are conducted, patients with full-thickness puncture wounds (i.e., completely penetrating the dermis into the subcutaneous tissue layers), full-thickness wounds of the hand or lower extremity, and dog bites that require surgical débridement should be considered at higher risk for infection and prescribed prophylactic antibiotic agents (Table 12–3). **Antibiotic agents effective against *Staphylococcus aureus* and *Pasteurella***

TABLE 12–2. INDICATIONS FOR ANTIBIOTIC ADMINISTRATION FOR ANIMAL BITE WOUNDS

Wound Factors

- Deep puncture wounds
- Extensive crush injury
- Involvement of underlying tendons or muscle
- Penetration into joint spaces
- Underlying fractures
- Retained foreign bodies

Patient Factors

- Risks factors for infective endocarditis (e.g., prosthetic valves, cardiac defects)
- Orthopedic prostheses
- Lymphedematous tissue
- Immunocompromise

TABLE 12–3. ANTIBIOTIC RECOMMENDATIONS FOR PROPHYLACTIC OR OUTPATIENT TREATMENT OF ANIMAL BITE WOUNDS

Bite	Primary	Alternative
Dog	Prophylaxis: Dicloxacillin or cephalexin 500 mg qid Infection (< 24 hours): Penicillin 500 mg qid Infection (> 24 hours): Dicloxacillin 500 mg qid	Azithromycin, clarithromycin, or fluoroquinolone (adults only)
Cat	Penicillin 500 mg qid or amoxicillin 500 mg tid	Cefuroxime axetil or doxycycline
Human	Penicillin 500 mg qid plus Dicloxacillin 500 mg qid	Clindamycin, fluoroquinolone, TMP-SMX, clarithromycin or azithromycin.
Pig	Penicillin 500 mg qid	Amoxicillin/clavulanic acid
Rat	Pencillin 500 mg qid	Doxycycline, erythromycin, clindamycin
Raccoon, skunk or bat	Pencillin 500 mg qid	Doxycycline

qid = four times a day; tid = three times a day; TMP-SMX = trimethoprim-sulfamethoxazole.

multocida **are efficacious for infection prophylaxis and should be administered for 3 to 5 days.**

If clinical signs of infection develop within 24 hours after the dog bite has occurred, the pathogen is probably *Pasteurella multocida*, but wound cultures should be obtained. Pencillin or amoxicillin can be used as initial antibiotic therapy to provide broad coverage. An initial intravenous (IV) or intramuscular (IM) dose of penicillin G, cefuroxime, or ceftriaxone can be administered in the emergency department before initiating outpatient oral therapy. Some authors recommend prescribing amoxicillin with clavulanic acid for its broad-spectrum coverage; however, it has a higher cost and a higher incidence of side effects, and no clinical studies have supported its use over other antibiotic agents.

Patients who develop clinical signs of wound infection more than 24 hours after a dog bite are more likely to have infections from *Staphylococcus* and *Streptococcus* spp. For this reason, an antistaphylococcal penicillin such as dicloxacillin or a first-generation cephalosporin should be used initially. In patients allergic to both penicillin and cephalosporins, azithromycin or clarithromycin should be used; in nonpregnant adults, tetracycline or a fluoroquinolone can also be used.

Low-risk patients with only local cellulitis and no deep structure involvement can be closely followed as outpatients. Patients with lymphangitis, lymphadenitis, tenosynovitis, septic arthritis, or systemic signs such as fever are best admitted for IV antibiotic therapy and surgical consultation.

Before wound culture results are received, initial inpatient antibiotic therapy for dog bite wound infections includes penicillin and nafcillin in those without sepsis, or imipenem-cilastatin or ampicillin/sulbactam if sepsis is suspected. This combination is acceptable for almost all patients, especially those with infections from *Pasteurella*, *Streptococcus*, or *Staphylococcus* spp. If gram-negative organisms are suspected or found, an aminoglycoside such as gentamycin should be added. Aerobic and anaerobic wound and blood cultures should be obtained when sepsis is suspected.

CAT BITES

Cat bites account for only 5 to 18 percent of all animal bites treated in emergency departments, even though there are as many cats as dogs in the United States.[8,16] Approximately 90 percent of patients who present to an emergency department after cat attacks have only one bite injury.[6,8] The most frequent complication is wound infection. Other complications such as sepsis, septic arthritis, tenosynovitis, fractures, osteomyelitis, peritonitis, endophthalmitis, meningitis, and disfiguring wounds may be seen.

Most (60 percent to 67 percent) cat bite injuries occur on the arm, forearm, or hands; 15 to 20 percent occur on the head and neck, 10 to 13 percent on the lower extremities, and no more than 5 percent occur on the trunk.[8] Puncture wounds are seen in 57 to 86 percent of cat bites, superficial abrasions in 9 to 25 percent, and lacerations in 5 to 17 percent.[8]

The bacteriology of cat bite wounds is perhaps less complex than other bites. The feline oral flora are more likely to contain *Pasteurella multocida*,[20,26] and this is the major pathogen in wound infections caused by cat bites.[7,8,16,21,26] This organism is carried in the oral or nasal secretions of 70 to 90 percent of cats,[21] and it is isolated in 53 to 80 percent of cultured cat bite wound infections.[7,8,16,20] *Staphylococcus aureus* wound infections are less common after cat bites than after dog bites.[8] Organisms recovered from cat bite wounds are listed in Table 12–1.

Cat bite victims with special conditions listed in Table 12–2 should be prescribed antibiotic agents. It is also recommended that patients who present with uninfected cat bites be prescribed antibiotics if they have full-thickness puncture wounds, hand or lower extremity wounds, or are older than age 50 years. **Antibiotic agents effective against *Pasteurella multocida* are efficacious for infection prophylaxis and should be administered for 3 to 5 days.**

Some clinicians recommend that the first dose of antibiotics should be administered parenterally, but there are no supporting data. Recommended prophylactic antibiotics are shown in Table 12–3. Just as for dog bites, patients with infections caused by cat bites should be treated based on how soon the clinical signs developed. Table 12–4 summarizes the recommended antibiotic agents and their dosages for the treatment of patients who have infected animal bites.

HUMAN BITES

Human bites are believed to be the third most frequent mammalian bite in the United States, but there is no estimate of the annual incidence. Hands are in-

TABLE 12–4. ANTIBIOTICS USED FOR LOCAL BITE WOUND INFECTIONS

Agents	Adult Dosage	Pediatric Dosage
Oral*		
Amoxicillin	500 mg tid	40 mg/kg per day divided into 3 doses
Amoxacillin/clavulanic acid	875 mg bid	
Azithromycin	500 mg stat, then 250 mg daily on days 2–5	10 mg/kg as a single dose on the first day (not to exceed 500 mg per day) followed by 5 mg/kg on days 2–5 (not to exceed 250 mg per day)
Cephalexin	250–500 mg qid	25–50 mg/kg per day divided into 4 doses
Clarithromycin	500 mg bid	7.5 mg/kg bid
Clindamycin	150–300 mg qid	8–16 mg/kg per day divided into 3 or 4 doses
Dicloxacillin	250–500 mg qid	12.5–50 mg/kg per day divided into 4 doses
Erythromycin	250–500 mg qid	40 mg/kg per day divided into 4 doses
Levofloxacin	250–500 mg qid	Not recommended
Penicillin VK	500 mg qid	50 mg/kg per day in children < 40 kg, divided into 4 doses
Parenteral		
Ampicillin-sulbactam	1.5–3 g tid–qid	Not recommended
Cefazolin	1–2 g tid–qid	25–50 mg/kg per day divided into 3 or 4 doses
Ceftriaxone	1–2 g qd	50–75 mg/kg per day
Cefuroxime	1–2 g tid	50–100 mg/kg per day divided into 3 doses
Clindamycin	500 mg qd	20–40 mg/kg per day divided into 3 or 4 doses
Erythromycin	500 mg qd	Not recommended
Imipenem-cilastin	0.5–1 g q 6 hours	Not recommended
Levofloxacin	250-500 mg qd	Not recommended
Nafcillin	1–2 g q 4 hours	150 mg/kg per day divided into 4 doses

TABLE 12–4. ANTIBIOTICS USED FOR LOCAL BITE WOUND INFECTIONS (Continued)

Agents	Adult Dosage	Pediatric Dosage
Oxacillin	1–2 g q 4 hours	150 mg/kg per day divided into 4 doses
Penicillin G	1–2 million unit q 6 hours	100,000–200,000 unit/kg per day divided into 4 doses
Ticarcillin-clavulanate	3.1 g q 6 hours	Not recommended
Vancomycin	0.5–1 g bid	40 mg/kg per day divided into 2 to 4 doses

* Prescribe 7–10 days of therapy.

volved in 60 to 75 percent of cases.[17] Two types of human bites are seen: occlusional bites and clenched-fist injuries (also known as fight bites, closed-fist injuries, or knuckle-tooth wounds). Occlusional bites occur when the teeth are sunk into the skin, crushing the tissue and creating tooth marks, contusion, abrasions, lacerations, avulsions, or amputations. Clenched-fist injuries occur when the closed fist strikes the teeth of another person, usually during a fight. These are considered the most serious of all human bite injuries. They most often occur in young men and involve the fourth metacarpophalangeal (MCP) joint of the dominant hand. The wound is typically small (5 mm in length) and is initially not considered serious by the patient; therefore, diagnosis is often delayed, resulting in a high incidence of complications. Within hours, the hand may become painful and edematous, and a purulent exudate may be present. **Any small laceration over a dorsal MCP joint should always be considered a human bite until confirmed otherwise.**

In clenched-fist injuries, there are three important hand spaces that may be violated by the teeth and thus contain bacterial inoculum: (1) the dorsal subcutaneous space, (2) the subtendinous space (between the tendon and the capsule where the subtendinous bursa is found), and (3) the joint space. Additionally, the metacarpal head may be fractured and penetrated. All clenched-fist injuries should undergo careful local exploration to rule out involvement of deeper structures. Because the injury occurs while the hand is clenched, the site of skin penetration moves proximal to the metacarpal head if the hand is extended during wound exploration. Thus, a partially injured tendon is usually retracted proximally from the wound, so the metacarpal head, joint capsule, and tendon seen just beneath the wound appear deceptively normal. To avoid failing to diagnose a joint capsule or tendon injury, the wound must be explored with the patient's hand in the clenched-fist position and throughout the entire range of motion.

Human bites in children are different from those in adults. Most are trivial, but some may result in serious complications.[27,28] Bitten children are most often engaged in fighting (62 percent), playing (26 percent), affectionate behavior (7 percent), sports (5 percent), or are victims of child abuse (1 percent).[10]

Most of the wounds (75 percent) are superficial abrasions that do not usually develop wound infection even if antibiotic agents are not prescribed.[10]

The most frequent complication of human bites is infection, including cellulitis, lymphangitis, and abscess. Farmer[29] reported a 50 percent incidence of infection after hand bites. These infections included osteomyelitis (16 percent), septic arthritis (12 percent), and tenosynovitis (22 percent).

BACTERIOLOGY

The most commonly cultured organisms from human bite wound infections are *Staphylococcus aureus* and *Streptococcus* spp.[10,30] Pure gram-negative infections in human bite wounds are uncommon.[30] They tend to follow in the wake of developing gram-positive infection, with little ability to establish infection alone. Anaerobic organisms appear in 42 percent of infected wounds, with the most common being *Enterobacter*, *Proteus*, *Serrati*, and *Eikenella* spp.[31]

Eikenella corrodens, a gram-negative rod that is a facultative anaerobe, is reported to be the infecting organism in 7 to 29 percent of human bites and is more common in clenched-fist injuries.[32] The organism is resistant to oxacillin, methicillin, nafcillin, most aminoglycosides, and clindamycin. It is sensitive to penicillin G, ampicillin, carbenicillin, cefoxitin, fluoroquinolones, trimethoprim-sulfamethoxazole, and tetracycline.[31,32] *Eikenella corrodens* is an important cause of chronic infection and should be suspected in patients treated with first-generation cephalosporins who do not respond to antibiotics.

PRESENTATION

Human bite wound infections of the hand present in two different ways: early (within 24 hours) or late (after more than 24 hours). Early patients present either after a clenched-fist injury or a bite with localized signs of infection, but they have normal erythrocyte sedimentation rates and white blood cell counts. Late patients present with considerable swelling, severe hand pain, and signs of cellulitis. Lymphangitis and fever may be present, a mild leukocytosis is seen, and a moderately profuse amount of malodorous exudate may be present. Tendon injury, septic arthritis, osteomyelitis, and tenosynovitis are significantly more common in those presenting late.[31] Radiographs of the hand are necessary to evaluate for fractures, foreign bodies, and osteomyelitis, although changes consistent with osteomyelitis usually are not evident for 7 to 10 days.

ANTIBIOTICS

Prophylactic antibiotics are not recommended for superficial wounds in children, but they should be prescribed for any patient with full-thickness wounds, particularly clenched-fist injuries and wounds that contain devitalized tissue. Specific recommendations are shown in Table 12–3.

Infected wounds should be cultured. Empiric antibiotics should include coverage for *Staphylococcus aureus*, *Eikenella corrodens*, *Haemophilus* spp., and anaerobic bacteria. Patients with infected hand wounds, immunodeficiency, or septic complications (e.g., lymphangitis, septic arthritis, or osteomyelitis) should be admitted. For inpatient therapy, the combination of penicillin G plus nafcillin or a first-generation cephalosporin is recommended. This regimen provides coverage for staphylococci, streptococci, and most anaerobes (including *Eikenella* spp.). Outpatients should be prescribed either penicillin plus dicloxacillin or cefuroxime for 3 to 5 days for infection prophylaxis or longer for established infections. Those allergic to penicillins and cephalosporins can be given clindamycin, a fluoroquinolone, trimethoprim-sulfamethoxazole, azithromycin, or clarithromycin. Patients should be re-evaluated every 36 to 48 hours until the infection is resolved.

LOCAL WOUND CARE OF ANIMAL BITES

Most bite wounds are minor, and local wound care begins with a thorough evaluation of the injury. The location, number, type, and depth of the wounds and any overt signs of wound infection should be assessed and documented. **Because bite wounds are frequently punctures, they are notoriously deceptive and may be more extensive than they appear.**

Evaluate for injuries of deeper structures such as tendons, joint spaces, blood vessels, nerves, and bone. Use local or regional anesthetic to facilitate wound exploration. A proximal tourniquet is used when appropriate to create a bloodless field. **If there is a considerable amount of edema and tenderness around the wound and bony penetration or foreign bodies are suspected, radiographs should be taken.** Subcutaneous emphysema may occasionally be noted on physical examination or seen on radiographs. This may represent gas from necrotizing infections or air introduced during wound manipulations. More often, however, it occurs when the animal holds on to the victim long enough to "grunt" or "snort" into the wound.

Meticulous wound cleansing, irrigation, and débridement are fundamental for the care of bite wounds. Because of the potential for disease transmission (e.g., rabies from animals; hepatitis and HIV from humans), a virucidal agent such as 1% povidone-iodine solution should be used during wound cleaning (Table 12–5). It remains to be determined whether one should attempt to irrigate bite puncture wounds. Their small cutaneous openings do not allow the solution to adequately drain out, and attempts at irrigation may result in infiltration. No clinical studies to date have compared excising or incising bite puncture wounds with enhanced irrigation.

Surgical débridement of wounds with a scalpel removes compromised or necrotic tissue that may contain embedded organisms, soil, and clots that cannot be removed by mechanical cleaning methods. Most bite wound lacerations contain crushed tissue and are not tidy lacerations. After wound débridement is performed, the wound should again be irrigated to remove any remaining contamination.

The question about whether to perform primary closure of dog bite wounds is controversial. The prevailing thought for many years was not to close most dog bite wounds. However, more recent investigations[4,6,14,21,34] support closure. Guy and Zook[4] reported 145 head and neck wounds inflicted by dogs. The wounds underwent primary closure; without antibiotics, the wound infection rate was only 1.4 percent. This supports the recommendation against the use

TABLE 12–5. BITE WOUND CLEANING PROTOCOL

1. Scrub the skin surrounding the bite wound with an antiseptic skin cleanser (e.g. Betadine® scrub, Hebiclens®, pHisoHex®), surfactant (Shur Clens®), or 1% povidone-iodine solution, with care not to allow the agent to contact the depth of the wound.
2. *(Optional)* Anesthetize the wound with a field block using a small-gauge hypodermic needle and a buffered local anesthetic (e.g., lidocaine, bupivacaine) or proceed to the next step.
3. Irrigate the wound with 1% povidone-iodine using a 20-mL syringe and a 20-gauge needle or IV catheter. Alternately, use a 20- to 35-mL syringe and a Zerowet® plastic shield (Zerowet, Inc., Palos Verdes, Calif.). Use 100 to 200 mL of irrigant for each 1 inch of wound length. Use a sterile skin hook or equivalent to retract the skin edges so the entire wound depth is adequately exposed and irrigated.
4. Anesthetize the wound edges using a 27- to 30-gauge hypodermic needle passed through the wound if a field block was not performed as described in Step 2.
5. Scrub the depth of the wound using a fine-pore sponge (e.g., Optipore®; Calgon-Vestal, St. Louis, Mo.) and 1% povidone-iodine solution.
6. Irrigate again as per Step 3.
7. Perform wound débridement, if indicated, using a no. 15 scalpel blade.
8. Irrigate again as per Step 3.
9. Cover the wound with a sterile gauze sponge until wound closure; or pack sterile, saline-soaked, fine-mesh gauze into the wound and apply a bandage cover if delayed primary closure is required.

of antibiotics, even when facial dog bite wounds are repaired in the emergency department.[6,33] Bite wound lacerations (> 1.5 cm in length) to the face or ears may be primarily repaired with sutures.[8] Small wounds (< 1.5 cm) behave as puncture wounds and should be kept open to allow for drainage. Chen and colleagues[34] found that carefully selected mammalian bite wounds that were closed primarily had approximately double the infection rate of other types of wounds (6 percent vs. 3 percent). Nevertheless, 94 percent of the bites that were closed did not develop any infection. Patients with wounds that require reconstructive surgery should be urgently referred to the appropriate specialist. Most hand wounds should be managed without immediate wound closure, but for cosmetic reasons, most facial wounds should be repaired primarily.[34] Delayed primary closure techniques may be used for other bite lacerations. Injured extremities should be immobilized and elevated.

TETANUS AND RABIES

Do not forget to address the need for tetanus and rabies immunoprophylaxis. Bites should be considered tetanus-prone wounds. Tetanus prophylaxis should be administered, as discussed in Chapter 17.

All victims of bites by both wild and domestic animals should be assessed for the need for rabies postexposure immunoprophylaxis. The recommendations by the Advisory Committee on Immunization Practices (ACIP) on Human Rabies Prevention—United States, 1999[35] (Table 12–6) should be followed, and local and state public health officials should be consulted. The incidence of rabies is highest in bats, raccoons, and skunks. In contrast, rodents and lagomorphs (e.g., rabbits and hares) rarely harbor rabies. Children and mentally limited individuals who have slept in a room where a bat was found should receive rabies prophylaxis even if no contact between the patient and the bat is known to have occurred.

Postexposure rabies immunoprophylaxis should include human diploid cell vaccine (HDCV) 1 mL IM on days 1, 3, 7, 14, and 28. It is given in the anterior

1, 3, 7, 14 ¿ 28 (5 shots)

TABLE 12–6. RABIES POSTEXPOSURE PROPHYLAXIS GUIDE, UNITED STATES, 1999

Animal Type	Evaluation and Disposition of Animal	Postexposure Prophylaxis Recommendations
Dogs, cats, and ferrets	Healthy and available for 10 days' observation	Patients should not begin prophylaxis unless animal develops clinical signs of rabies*
	Rabid or suspected rabid	Immediately vaccinate
	Unknown (e.g., escaped)	Consult public health officials
Skunks, raccoons, foxes, and most other carnivores; bats	Regarded as rabid unless animal proven negative by laboratory tests[†]	Consider immediate vaccination
Livestock, small rodents, lagomorphs (rabbits and hares), large rodents (woodchucks and beavers), and other mammals	Consider individually	Consult public health officials Bites of squirrels, hamsters, guinea pigs, gerbils, chipmunks, rats, mice, other small rodents, rabbits, and hares almost never require antirabies postexposure prophylaxis

Reprinted from Talan, DA, and Moran, GJ: Update on emerging infections from the Centers for Disease Control and Prevention. Ann Emerg Med 33:592, 1999, with permission.

*During the 10-day observation period, begin postexposure prophylaxis at the first sign of rabies in a dog, cat, or ferret that has bitten someone. If the animal exhibits clinical signs of rabies, it should be euthanized immediately and tested.

[†]The animal should be euthanized and tested as soon as possible. Holding for observation is not recommended. Discontinue vaccine if immunofluorescence test results of the animal are negative.

thigh of children and the deltoid muscle of adults. Passive immunization with 20 IU/kg of human rabies immune globulin (HRIG) is also administered. Half of the dose is infiltrated around the wound site, and the rest is given IM in the gluteal muscle.

Rabies IG : 20 iu/kg — 1/2 in wound
1/2 in deltoid
or gluteus

REFERENCES

1. Weiss, HB, Friedman, DI, and Coben, JH: Incidence of dog bite injuries treated in emergency departments. JAMA 279:51–53, 1998.
2. Callaham, M: Prophylactic antibiotics in common dog bite wounds: A controlled study. Ann Emerg Med 9:410–414, 1980.
3. Goldstein, EJC, Citron, DM, and Finegold, SM: Dog bite wounds and infection: A prospective clinical study. Ann Emerg Med 9:508–512, 1980.
4. Guy, RJ, and Zook, EG: Successful treatment of acute head and neck dog bite wounds without antibiotics. Ann Plastic Surg 17:45–48, 1986.
5. Palmer, J, and Rees, M: Dog bite of the face: A 15-year review. Br J Plastic Surg 36:315–318, 1983.
6. Dire, DJ, Hogan, DE, and Riggs, MW: A prospective evaluation of risk factors for infection from dog-bite wounds. Acad Emerg Med 1:258–266, 1994.
7. Elenbaas, RM, McNabney, WK, and Robinson, WA: Evaluation of prophylactic oxacillin in cat bite wounds. Ann Emerg Med 13:155–157, 1984.
8. Dire, DJ: Cat bite wounds: risk factors for infection. Ann Emerg Med 19:973–979, 1991.
9. Schweich, P, and Fleischer, G: Human bites in children. Pediatr Emerg Care 1:51–53, 1985.
10. Baker, MD, and Moore, SE: Human bites in children: A six-year experience. Am J Dis Child 141:1285–1290, 1987.
11. Lindsey, D, Christopher, M, Hollenbach, J, et al: Natural course of the human bite wound: Incidence of infection and complications in 434 bites and 803 lacerations in the same group of patients. J Trauma 27:45–48, 1987.
12. Dire, DJ, Hogan, DE, and Walker, JS: Prophylactic oral antibiotics for low risk dog bite wounds. Pediatr Emerg Care 8:194–199, 1992.
13. Wiley, JF: Mammalian bites: Review of evaluation and management. Clin Pediatr 29:283–287, 1990.
14. Karlson, TA: The incidence of facial injuries from dog bites. JAMA 251:3265–3267, 1984.
15. Thomas, PR, and Buntine, JA: Man's best friend?: A review of the Austin Hospital's experience with dog bites. Med J Austral 147:536–540, 1987.
16. Aghababian, RV, and Conte, JE: Mammalian bite wounds. Ann Emerg Med 9:79–83, 1980.
17. Goldstein, EJC, Citron, DM, Wield, B, et al: Bacteriology of human and animal bite wounds. J Clin Microbiol 8:667–672, 1978.
18. Bailie, WE, Stowe, EC, and Schmitt, AM: Aerobic bacterial flora of oral and nasal fluids of canines with reference to bacteria associated with bites. J Clin Microbiol 7:223-231, 1978.
19. Ganiere, JP, Escande, F, Andre, G, et al: Characterization of Pasteurella from gingival scrapings of dogs and cats. Comp Immuno Microbiol Infect Dis 16:77–85, 1993.
20. Talan, DA, Citron, DM, Abrahamian, FM, et al: Bacteriologic analysis of infected dog and cat bites. Emergency Medicine Animal Bite Infection Study Group. N Engl J Med 340:85–92, 1999.
21. Weber, DJ, Wolfson, JS, Swartz, MN, et al: Pasteurella multocida infections: Report of 34 cases and review of the literature. Medicine 63:133–154, 1984.
22. Goldstein, EJC, and Citron, DM: Comparative activities of cefuroxime, amoxacillin-clavulanic acid, ciprofloxacin, enoxacin, and ofloxacin against aerobic and anaerobic bacteria isolated from bite wounds. Antimicrob Agents Chemother 32:1143–1147, 1988.
23. Goldstein, EJC, Citron, DM, Gerardo, SH, et al: Activities of HMR 3004 (RU 64004) and HMR 3647 (RU 66647) compared to those of erythromycin, azithromycin, clarithromycin, roxithromycin, and eight other antimicrobial agents against unusual aerobic and anaerobic human and animal bite pathogens isolated from skin and soft tissue infections in humans. Antimicrob Agents Chemother 42:1127–1132, 1998.
24. Cummings, P: Antibiotics to prevent infection in patients with dog bite wounds: A meta-analysis of randomized trials. Ann Emerg Med 23:535–540, 1994.

25. Callaham, M: Prophylactic antibiotics in dog bite wounds: Nipping at the heels of progress. Ann Emerg Med 23:577–579, 1994.
26. Feder, HM, Shanley, JD, and Barbera, JA: Review of 59 patients hospitalized with animal bites. Pediatr Infect Dis J 6:24–28, 1987.
27. Schweich, P, and Fleischer, G: Human bites in children. Pediatr Emerg Care 1:51–53, 1985.
28. Leung, AKC, and Robson, WLM: Human bites in children. Pediatr Emerg Care 8:255–257, 1992.
29. Farmer, CB, and Mann, RJ: Human bite infections of the hand. South Med J 59:515–518, 1966.
30. Zubowicz, VN, and Gravier, M: Management of early human bites of the hand: A prospective randomized study. Plast Reconstruct Surg 88:111–114, 1991.
31. Basadre, JO, and Parry, SW: Indications for surgical debridement in 125 human bites to the hand. Arch Surg 126:65–67, 1991.
32. Faciszewski, T, and Coleman, DA: Human bite wounds. Hand Clin 5:561–569, 1989.
33. Callaham, M: Controversies in antibiotic choices for bite wounds. Ann Emerg Med 17:1321–1330, 1988.
34. Chen, E, Hornig, S, Sheperd, SM, et al: Primary closure of mammalian bite wounds. Acad Emerg Med 7:157–161, 2000.
35. Centers for Disease Control and Prevention: Human rabies prevention—United States, 1999. Recommendations of the Advisory Committee on Immunization Practices (ACIP). MMWR Morb Mortal Wkly Rep 48 (No. RR-1):1–21, 1999.

RICHARD LAMMERS, MD

CHAPTER

13

Foreign Bodies in Wounds

Only a small percentage of lacerations and puncture wounds treated in emergency departments contain foreign bodies, but physicians must consider the possibility of a concealed foreign body in any wound that penetrates the dermis. **All wounds should be explored for concealed foreign bodies.** Some foreign bodies are serendipitously discovered in wounds, but most are found during deliberate, careful searches in wounds that are considered high risk. **Most foreign bodies can be found by wound exploration or imaging studies, but not all foreign bodies are accessible.** All accessible foreign material within new lacerations should be irrigated away, débrided, or extracted with instruments. However, not all foreign bodies embedded within soft tissue require removal. The decision to remove a deeper foreign body depends on its size, location, composition, accessibility, and anticipated mechanical and inflammatory effects.

Various imaging studies can be used to evaluate wounds when the history or physical examination suggests the presence of a retained foreign body even though nothing is found during exploration. However, some of the most harmful types of foreign bodies may not be visible with any type of radiographic or sonographic study.

PATHOPHYSIOLOGY

Reactive foreign bodies should be removed before severe inflammation or infection develop. When reactive foreign bodies are left in a wound, the normal inflammatory response during wound healing may intensify and can delay healing or destroy the surrounding soft tissue and bone. The type and intensity of an inflammatory reaction is primarily determined by the chemical composition and physical form of the foreign object.[1] Whereas material that is inert (e.g., glass, metal, or plastic) may not elicit any abnormal tissue response, vegetative foreign bodies provoke intense inflammation. Objects with smooth,

147

nonporous surfaces produce less inflammation and fibrosis than those with rough surfaces. If the body fails to dissolve or extrude foreign material, it may encapsulate it within a cyst. After a retained foreign body is encapsulated, inflammation subsides.[1]

Infection is the most common complication. All foreign substances in soft tissue increase the risk of soft tissue and bone infections, including local wound infection, cellulitis, abscess formation, lymphangitis, tenosynovitis, bursitis, arthritis, synovitis, and osteomyelitis.[1–4] Infection may develop even when the foreign material itself is not contaminated. Sterile foreign bodies implanted in the subcutaneous tissues of guinea pigs lowered the threshold for local infection when bacteremia was induced.[5]

Foreign objects can cause mechanical damage by compressing or lacerating anatomical structures, sometimes years after the initial injury.[6,7] Some authors[8] have reported on foreign bodies that have resulted in vascular occlusion, erosion, thrombus formation, or migration to distant sites. Repeated movement of tissue that contains a foreign object increases the fibrous reaction. Mechanical complications of foreign bodies are listed in Table 13–1.

CLINICAL EVALUATION

Information obtained from a patient's history and physical examination may suggest the presence of foreign bodies (Table 13–2). The mechanism of injury and shape of the wounding object help determine the type of foreign body, its depth, and the likelihood of multiple fragments. Bites, clenched-fist injuries, and intraoral lacerations may contain tooth fragments. Objects that shatter, splinter, or break when inflicting a wound often leave behind remnants. Wood splinters tend to fragment when they are pulled out of a puncture wound. Thin needles, thorns, and spines often deeply penetrate soft tissue before breaking off. When glass has broken in an individual's hand, a higher risk of a glass foreign body exists than if previously broken glass lacerates skin. In a study[9] with a 7 percent prevalence of glass in wounds, puncture wounds were more likely to contain glass than were lacerations. Lacerations sustained when a forehead impacts a windshield have a high chance of hiding multiple glass fragments.[10]

TABLE 13–1. POTENTIAL MECHANICAL COMPLICATIONS RESULTING FROM RETAINED FOREIGN BODIES

- Laceration of vessels, nerves, and tendons
- Occlusion of vessels with distal ischemia
- Erosion of vessels
- Compression of vessels
- Migration
- Embolization
- Persistent pain
- Impaired function
- Fibrous reaction

TABLE 13–2. HIGH-RISK FINDINGS SUGGESTIVE OF A FOREIGN BODY

History

- Mechanism of injury
  - Glass breaking on skin vs. sharp glass lacerating skin
  - Blunt oral trauma with tooth fragments
  - Clenched-fist injuries
  - Missile injuries
  - Pneumatic nail guns (epidermal inclusion cyst)
  - High-pressure injection guns
- Shape of wounding object
- Sharp pain with movement or pressure
- Infected puncture wound
- Infection resistant to antibiotics
- Failure to heal
- Persistent pain
- Chronic, delayed, and recurrent infections
- Arthritis near an old puncture wound
- Delayed nerve, vessel, or tendon injuries

Physical Examination

- Surface discoloration
- Palpable mass
- Sharp pain with palpation
- Grating or resistance
- Blood-stained tract
- Abscess formation
- Chronic draining sinus
- Sterile purulent drainage
- Fibrous or granulomatous tissue

If multiple pieces of glass are discovered in a wound, a radiograph should be obtained after débridement to confirm the removal of all pieces. Nails that are stepped on and penetrate shoes and socks may drive leather, rubber, or cloth into the plantar surface of a patient's foot.[4] Patients are not always aware of foreign bodies in their wounds, but a patient's sensation of "something in the wound" should be taken seriously; these perceptions are frequently correct.[9,10] Sharp, well-localized pain with palpation over a puncture wound is a useful sign.

WOUND EXPLORATION

All lacerations should be visually inspected for foreign bodies. Adequate lighting, good hemostasis, complete local anesthesia, and patient cooperation are essential for success. Because puncture wounds are narrow and deep, they are more difficult to examine. If a physician is concerned that a puncture wound contains a foreign body, the wound margins can be extended with a scalpel.

Blind probing of deep wounds with a closed hemostat may produce a grating sensation if a hard object is contacted, but failure to feel foreign bodies with probing does not exclude them.[10] The instrument should not be used to grasp blindly for potential foreign objects. Because this technique can result in damage to underlying structures, it is especially dangerous to use it in wounds that involve the hands, feet, and face. In most situations, direct visualization is the preferred method of exploration. **Sometimes the damage caused by an attempt to locate a foreign body is not worth the benefit provided by its removal.**

DIAGNOSTIC IMAGING STUDIES

Imaging studies of acute wounds should be considered if a wound foreign body is suspected but is not found during wound exploration; multiple foreign bodies are removed but some pieces may have been missed; the object may have fragmented during removal; or thorough wound exploration is technically impossible.

Several types of imaging studies are available. The advantages and disadvantages of each one are listed in Table 13–3. The size, shape, density, and orientation relative to the imaging beam determine whether an object is visible. The physician should select a study on the basis of the density of the suspected object. Many foreign bodies commonly found in wounds are much denser than the surrounding tissue and are readily apparent on plain radiographs.[11] Computed tomography (CT) and magnetic resonance imaging (MRI) are useful for identifying and locating objects that have densities similar to soft tissue. Materials that are the same density as surrounding soft tissue are difficult to see with any type of radiographic or sonographic technique.

Plain Radiography

Of all the imaging studies used, plain radiography is the most readily available, easiest to interpret, and least expensive. **Many foreign bodies are radiopaque, so plain radiography can be used as a screening study in high-risk patients. Plain radiographs should be ordered if a patient reports a sensation of a retained foreign body.** Metal, bone, teeth, pencil graphite, certain plastics, glass, gravel, sand, some fish bones, some wood, and some aluminum are visible on plain radiographs.[12–14] Almost all glass is visible on radiographs if it is 2 mm or larger. More than half of glass fragments between 0.5 and 2.0 mm in size can be seen.[13] Glass does not have to contain lead to be visible on plain radiographs.[15] A small fragment of glass is more easily seen if it is positioned parallel to the central ray of the x-ray beam, increasing the apparent thickness of the fragment. The contrast between foreign bodies and the surrounding tissue is enhanced in underpenetrated radiographs compared with radiographs taken using the standard technique.[16] If the wound was caused by metal or glass and no foreign body was found on wound exploration or on a plain radiograph, it is unlikely that a foreign body exists. However, radiopaque foreign bodies may be invisible on plain radiographs if they are embedded within bone or overlie bones in all projections.

TABLE 13–3. COMPARISON OF IMAGING MODALITIES

Imaging Modality	Advantages	Disadvantages
Plain radiography	Readily available Easy to interpret Shows most foreign bodies	Two-dimensional Vegetative material not visible
Fluoroscopy	Real-time exploration Improved positioning by rotation	Radiation exposure Use restricted
CT	Sensitivity in differentiating densities Shows a variety of materials Shows the relationship of the object to anatomical structures	More costly than other methods More radiation than other methods
Ultrasonography	No radiation Real-time exploration Readily available in some centers	Numerous artifacts, including residual air in wound
MRI	May be more sensitive than CT Shows greater variety of materials Shows the relationship of the object to anatomical structures No radiation	More costly than other methods Must exclude the possibility of metallic foreign bodies Inadequately studied

It is usually easier to detect the presence of a foreign body than to locate its exact position in the tissue. The depth and position of radiopaque foreign bodies can be estimated by taking plain radiographs in multiple projections. If radiopaque skin markers such as lead circles, paperclips, or hypodermic needles are placed around the wound entrance, the position of the object can be estimated relative to these surface landmarks. To remove the object, an incision can be made between needles or markers or dissection can be carried along the path of the closest needle.[17,18] However, multiple projections do not provide a true three-dimensional image, and tendons and other important structures that are invisible on plain radiographs may block the most accessible path to the foreign body.

Fluoroscopy

Fluoroscopy is used primarily for locating foreign bodies during removal, but bedside imagers are sometimes used to identify their presence. Accurate localization of a foreign body before its removal is important because blind searching is time consuming and can cause further injury. The site of injury can be rotated under fluoroscopy to visualize the object between surface markers.

Radiation exposure should be minimized by brief, intermittent imaging and appropriate shielding.

Computed Tomography

Computed tomography is capable of detecting more types of foreign material than plain film radiography because it is 100 times more sensitive in differentiating densities, particularly with a narrow window adjustment and with digital edge-enhancement techniques.[16,19,20] Some wood, thorns, and spines not visible on plain radiographs have been identified with this method,[19,20] but not all types are visible.[11] CT images can be created in multiple planes and can demonstrate the relationship of a foreign object to important anatomical structures. Isodense objects may be outlined by surrounding air within the wound, producing a radiolucent filling defect.

Ultrasonography

Sonography has been used with variable success to diagnose soft tissue foreign bodies in experimental models. Some investigators have accurately identified wood, fish bones, sea urchin spines, and other vegetative materials; however, for other investigators, the false-positive rate for nonradiopaque foreign bodies is excessive. In various studies,[21-23] the overall sensitivity of ultrasonography ranged from 50 to 90 percent and the specificity ranged from 70 to 97 percent for gravel, metal, glass, cactus spines, wood, and plastic. The accuracy of this technique depends on the size of the object and the skill of the operator. Objects that produce echo artifacts include pockets of air, blood, calcifications, sesamoid bones, sutures, purulence, and old scar tissue.[24] Small objects that are oriented perpendicular to the skin surface or adjacent to tendons are more easily missed. Some areas of the body may not accommodate an ultrasound probe.

An advantage of sonography is that after the presence of a foreign body is confirmed, this technique can provide dynamic images in different axes that help guide an instrument to the object during retrieval. A 7.5-MHz linear-array transducer can be used to find objects as deep as 3 cm. The scanning beam should be oriented parallel to the long axis of a hemostat.[25]

Magnetic Resonance Imaging

The role of MRI for detection of foreign bodies in soft tissue is unclear at this time. It cannot be used if the foreign body contains metal or gravel. MRI may be more effective than CT in identifying vegetative foreign bodies such as wood, spines, and thorns, but comparative studies are needed.[26] MRI is usually reserved for situations in which plain radiography, ultrasonography, and CT fail to find an isodense object in a high-risk wound.

TREATMENT

DETERMINING IF AN OBJECT SHOULD BE REMOVED

When a foreign body is discovered in a wound, the physician must weigh the risk of leaving the foreign body in place against the potential harm of attempting to remove it. Not all foreign bodies must be removed, and not all that require removal must be extracted during the initial evaluation. Nevertheless, every effort should be made to identify their presence during the initial visit.

Indications for removal of foreign bodies from wounds are listed in Table 13–4. **Inert foreign bodies that are deep within tissues and not causing symptoms or injury to anatomical structures can be left in place.** Most foreign bodies in the hands, which are mobile and sensitive, should be removed. Bullets that are lodged within a muscle belly are ordinarily not removed because the procedure can cause more damage than leaving the bullet in place. Projectiles may drag bits of clothing or skin into the wound, however, so this foreign material should be removed.

Vegetative foreign bodies cause intense and excessive inflammation and should be removed immediately. Foreign objects that are heavily contaminated, such as fractured teeth and soil-covered objects, should be removed as soon as possible, and the patient should be treated expectantly with antibiotics. Glass, metal, and plastic are relatively inert, and removal can be

TABLE 13–4. INDICATIONS FOR FOREIGN BODY REMOVAL

Potential for Inflammation or Infection

- Vegetative or chemically reactive material
- Heavy bacterial contamination (e.g., teeth, soil)
- Proximity to fractured bone
- Established infection
- Allergic reaction

Functional and Cosmetic Problems

- Impingement on nerves, vessels, or tendons
- Restriction of joint mobility
- Proximity to tendons
- Impairment of gait
- Persistent pain
- Cosmetic deformity (e.g., tattooing)
- Psychological distress

Potential for Later Injury

- Intra-articular location
- Intravascular location
- Migration toward important structures

Toxicity

- Spines with venom
- Heavy metals

Source: Reprinted with permission from Lammers, RL: Soft tissue foreign bodies. In Tintinalli JE, Kelen GD, Stapczynski JS (eds): Emergency Medicine: A Comprehensive Study Guide. McGraw-Hill, New York, 2000, p. 326.

postponed, if necessary. However, glass and other sharp foreign bodies in the hands or feet can cause persistent pain when the patient is gripping objects or walking, and they can sever nerves or tendons years after the initial injury.[6,7] Patients with deep foreign bodies in these locations should be referred to appropriate specialists for eventual removal. Pain, patient concern, psychological distress, and cosmetic problems are also indications for elective removal of inert foreign bodies.

REMOVAL PROCEDURES

Removal of foreign bodies requires local or regional anesthesia, good lighting, adequate hemostasis, patient cooperation, time, and sometimes magnification and assistance. Accessibility of the object and physician time are the usual limiting factors. Depending on circumstances in the emergency department or primary care setting, the physician may not be able to devote more than about 15 to 30 minutes to the removal procedure. Removal techniques include extraction by splinter or alligator forceps, dissection and débridement, and block excision.[27–30] **Do not forget to clean the wound after successful removal of a foreign body.**

If deep exploration is required, the procedure should be referred to a surgical specialist. Patients who are referred to surgical specialists for delayed removal of foreign bodies in any location should be told that the object is present but unlikely to cause harm before it is removed. **If the foreign body is near a joint or highly mobile region, splint the area to prevent further injury or migration before definitive removal.**

ANTIBIOTICS

The benefit of prophylactic antibiotics for retained foreign bodies has not been studied. Clinical experience suggests that infections in wounds that contain foreign bodies are resistant to antibiotics, but these infections often resolve spontaneously after the foreign bodies are removed.[26] Antibiotics seem justified for infected wounds, particularly when foreign body removal must be postponed, and for wounds in which foreign bodies penetrate bones, joints, or tendons.

DOCUMENTATION

Whatever decisions are made, patients should be informed of the presence of known retained foreign bodies, the potential for undiscovered foreign bodies, and the effects they may have on soft tissues. The essential components of charting wound management also apply to foreign body management. The physician should report one of the following strategies:

1. The wound was explored for foreign bodies and none were found, and the wound is at low risk for containing occult foreign bodies.

2. A high-risk wound was explored for foreign bodies and none were found, and additional imaging studies failed to demonstrate foreign bodies.
3. A foreign body was removed, the wound was re-explored, and no other foreign bodies were found.
4. A foreign body was identified by radiologic studies and a reasonable attempt to remove it failed, or no attempt was made and the patient was referred to a surgeon.
5. A foreign body was identified, but the physician chose to leave it in place because it was inaccessible and inert.

Damage caused by the foreign body, including inflammation, infection, and mechanical complications, should be documented. When a foreign body lies in proximity to nerves, vessels, and tendons, the physician should evaluate and document the function of these structures after foreign body removal.

REFERENCES

1. Hirsh, BC, and Johnson, WC: Pathology of granulomatous diseases: Foreign body granulomas. Int J Dermatol 23:531–538, 1984.
2. Brand, RA, and Black, H: Pseudomonas osteomyelitis following puncture wounds in children. J Bone Joint Surg 56(suppl A):1637–1642, 1974.
3. Strömqvist, B, Edlund, E, and Lidgren, L: A case of blackthorn synovitis. Acta Orthop Scand 56:342–343, 1985.
4. Riegler, HF, and Routson, GW: Complications of deep puncture wounds of the foot. J Trauma 19:18–22, 1979.
5. Zimmerli, W, Zak, O, and Vosbeck, K: Experimental hematogenous infection of subcutaneously implanted foreign bodies. Scand J Infect Dis 17:303–310, 1985.
6. Browett, JP, and Fiddian, NJ: Delayed median nerve injury due to retained glass fragments. J Bone Joint Surg 67:382–384, 1985.
7. Jablon, M, and Rabin, SI: Late flexor pollicis longus tendon rupture due to retained glass fragments. J Hand Surg 13(suppl A):713–716, 1988.
8. Dadsetan, MR, and Jinkins, JR: Peripheral vascular gunshot bullet embolus migration to the cerebral circulation: Report and literature review. Neuroradiology 36:516–519, 1990.
9. Montano, JB, Steele, MT, and Watson, WA: Foreign body retention in glass-caused wounds. Ann Emerg Med 21:1360–1363, 1992.
10. Steele, MT, Tran, LV, Watson, WA, et al: Retained glass foreign bodies in wounds: Predictive value of wound characteristics, patient perception, and wound exploration. Am J Emerg Med 16:627–630, 1998.
11. Lammers, RL: Soft tissue foreign bodies. Ann Emerg Med 17:1336–1347, 1988.
12. Ellis, G: Are aluminum foreign bodies detectable radiographically? Am J Emerg Med 11:12, 1993.
13. Courter, BJ: Radiographic screening for glass foreign bodies: What does a "negative" foreign body series really mean? Ann Emerg Med 19:997–1000, 1990.
14. Chisholm, CD, Wood, CO, Chua, G, et al: Radiographic detection of gravel in soft tissue. Ann Emerg Med 29:725–730, 1997.
15. Felman, AH, and Fisher, MS: The radiographic detection of glass in soft tissue. Radiology 92:1529–1531, 1969.
16. Roobottom, CA, and Weston, MJ: The detection of foreign bodies in soft tissue: Comparison of conventional and digital radiography. Clin Radiol May 49:330–332, 1994.
17. Gahhos, F, and Arons, MS: Soft-tissue foreign body removal: Management and presentation of a new technique. J Trauma 24:340–341, 1984.
18. Rickoff, SE, Bauder, T, and Kerman, BL: Foreign body localization and retrieval in the foot. J Foot Surg 20:33–34, 1981.
19. Kuhns, LR, Borlaza, GS, Seigel, RS, et al: An in vitro comparison of computed tomography, xerography, and radiography in the detection of soft-tissue foreign bodies. Radiology 132:218–219, 1979.

20. Bauer, AR, and Yutani, D: Computed tomographic localization of wooden foreign bodies in children's extremities. Arch Surg 118:1084–1086, 1983.
21. Hill, R, Conron, R, Greissinger, P, et al: Ultrasound for the detection of foreign bodies in human tissue. Ann Emerg Med 29:353–356, 1997.
22. Manthey, DE, Storrow, AB, Milbourn, JM, et al: Ultrasound versus radiography in the detection of soft-tissue foreign bodies. Ann Emerg Med 28:7–9, 1996.
23. Jacobson, JA, Powell, A, Craig, JG, et al: Wooden foreign bodies in soft tissue: Detection at ultrasound. Radiology 206:45–48, 1998.
24. Gilbert, FJ, Campbell, RSD, and Bayliss, AP: The role of ultrasound in the detection of non-radiopaque foreign bodies. Clin Radiol 41:109–112, 1990.
25. Shiels, WE, Babcock, DS, Wilson, JL, et al: Localization and guided removal of soft-tissue foreign bodies with sonography. Am J Roentgenol 155:1277–1281, 1990.
26. Bodne, D, Quinn, SF, and Cochran, CF: Imaging foreign glass and wooden bodies of the extremities with CT and MR. J Comput Assist Tomogr 12:608–611, 1988.
27. Gilsdorf, JR: A needle in the sole of the foot. Surg Gynecol Obstet 163:573–574, 1986.
28. Rees, CE: The removal of foreign bodies: A modified incision. JAMA 113:35, 1939.
29. Reinherz, RP, Hong, DT, and Tisa, LM: Management of puncture wounds in the foot. J Foot Surg 24:288–292, 1985.
30. Stein, F: Foreign body injuries of the hand. Emerg Med Clin North Am 3:383–390, 1985.

RICHARD LAMMERS, MD

Plantar Puncture Wounds

Physicians have widely divergent views on the management of plantar puncture wounds. Some prefer expectant therapy, reacting to complications as they develop. Others pursue potential foreign bodies with relatively invasive exploration, hoping to prevent unusual but devastating infections. **No clear evidence supports either an aggressive or conservative approach to the management of plantar puncture wounds, so the patient should be involved in the decision-making process.**

As with other injuries containing potential foreign bodies (see Chapter 13), infection is the most common complication. The principles of clinical evaluation, use of imaging studies, and the risks and benefits of exploration are discussed in Chapter 13. This chapter highlights certain areas of difference in the treatment and evaluation of puncture wounds, especially in the feet.

COMPLICATIONS OF PUNCTURE WOUNDS

The complication rate from plantar puncture wounds is higher than the rate for puncture wounds in the rest of the lower extremities. One reason for this is the small distance from the plantar skin surface to the bones and joints of the feet. Another reason is the force with which puncture wounds are inflicted as the weight of the body presses against a sharp object. Finally, penetration of a shoe and sock by a nail can push foreign bodies into the deepest recesses of the wound. This debris is seldom visible on plain radiographs.

Infections in these puncture wounds can have serious consequences and lead to lifetime disability or amputations. Osteomyelitis, osteochondritis, and septic arthritis are the most serious complications. *Staphylococcus aureus* and *Pseudomonas aeruginosa* are the most common isolates from plantar puncture wound infections.[1] Osteomyelitis caused by *Pseudomonas* spp. is associated with nail penetration of rubber-soled work boots or athletic shoes, probably because these organisms grow well in this environment and have a predilection for the cartilage in the foot.[2,3] Although uncommon, clostridial infections also can develop in deep, closed wounds such as those caused by nail punctures of the feet.

In a retrospective analysis of 2325 patients presenting to an emergency department with punctures, Houston and coworkers[4] reported a 2 percent infection rate with early treatment of these wounds and a 10 percent rate if patients presented late. The rate of osteomyelitis was 0.04 percent.

Fitzgerald and Cowan[1] reported a study of 887 puncture wounds in the feet, mostly in children: 98 percent of the wounds were caused by nails. Foreign bodies were found in 3 percent: 50 percent of them were pieces of shoe or sock, and 50 percent were rust, gravel, grass, straw, or dirt. Of the 774 patients who were treated in the emergency department within 24 hours, 8.4 percent either already had cellulitis or subsequently developed cellulitis. In the group of patients who presented for treatment 1 to 7 days after injury, 57 percent had cellulitis or a soft tissue infection. Almost 7 percent of the infections in these patients' puncture wounds failed to respond to antimicrobial therapy and required incision and drainage of an abscess. Of all the patients in this series, 4 percent developed serious infections, and osteomyelitis occurred in almost 2 percent. In some cases, osteomyelitis developed despite the use of antibiotics. *Pseudomonas* spp. was isolated in 81 percent of these infections.[1]

The risk of infection in all victims of puncture wounds of the feet is unknown because many people never seek medical care for these injuries. Weber[5] estimated this risk in a survey of 200 emergency department patients who were asked to recall their past experiences with plantar puncture wounds. Of these subjects, 44 percent reported puncturing their foot at some time during their life, and 50 percent of those had sought medical care for the injury. Ten subjects reported infections, nine of whom sought medical care. In this study, the infection rate in patients who had presented for treatment of plantar puncture wounds was 20.5 percent; in all patients with this injury, the infection rate was 11.4 percent. The author concluded that many wounds with a benign outcome never come to medical attention, so the infection rate from this injury is lower than reported.[5] Nevertheless, the self-reported infection rate was higher than in previous retrospective studies.

MANAGEMENT STRATEGIES

EXPLORATION

Blind probing of deep puncture wounds is especially dangerous in wounds that involve the hand, foot, or face because the probing can result in damage to underlying structures. In most situations, direct visualization is the preferred method of exploration. Exploration of any deep puncture wound for foreign bodies poses a technical challenge, but plantar puncture wounds present additional problems. The skin in this region is thick, relatively rigid, and quite sensitive. Foreign bodies that penetrate the plantar fascia are almost impossible to locate through a narrow wound. Even irrigation of deep puncture wounds is often futile because the irrigant solution does not completely drain out of the wound.

One of the unresolved controversies about plantar puncture wounds is whether to explore all of these wounds for foreign bodies; another is whether probing constitutes a sufficient exploration. Schwab and Powers[6] reported a 3 percent rate of retained foreign bodies after initial surface cleansing without wound exploration. Some authors[7] recommend enlarging the puncture wound to allow deeper exploration and irrigation, particularly if bone or joint contact is suspected.[8] Others[9] believe that excising a block or cone of tissue down to the subcutaneous layer—or "coring out" the wound with a punch biopsy—allows adequate visualization of accessible foreign bodies and removal of most of the contaminated tissue. Others simply trim jagged epidermal skin edges with a tissue scissors or scalpel.[10] Simple probing and blind grasping have unknown false-negative rates[11] and may force foreign objects deeper into the wound.[12]

It is not clear what percentage of unexpected foreign bodies are discovered and removed during the initial visit and how many infections may be averted as a result of probing, excising, or incising and exploring plantar puncture wounds. Healing of a puncture wound may be delayed somewhat by excising or incising the wound, but infection delays healing even more. It is recommended that clinicians extend the length of new, uninfected wounds and explore them by spreading wound edges apart if the punctures have been caused by thorns, spines, wood splinters, or contaminated objects (which present a very high risk for complications) or by nails that penetrate footwear (because these wounds frequently harbor accessible foreign bodies). If debris is visible in the wound tract, a small amount of tissue should be excised. Punctures caused by sewing needles do not require exploration, but plain radiographs should be used for patients with these types of wounds. Significant glass remnants also show on plain films. If infection is present, the risk of a foreign body is high and imaging or exploration is warranted.

Exploration of plantar puncture wounds can be quite painful. **Anesthesia is best achieved through the use of regional ankle blocks (see Chapter 4), with or without procedural sedation (see Chapter 5).**

ANTIBIOTIC AGENTS

Prophylactic antibiotic agents are recommended by some clinicians, but no studies prove a benefit. Many authors[2,3,12–14] recommend against the use of antibiotic therapy for new plantar puncture wounds, saying "antibiotics will not compensate for inadequate primary wound care," they are ineffective in wounds with retained foreign bodies, they may contribute to a gram-negative overgrowth, and subsequent infection responds quickly to the addition of antibiotics. The only study of antibiotic use in plantar puncture wounds was published by Pennycook and colleagues.[15] In this nonrandomized, uncontrolled observational study, the use of antibiotic agents was optional, and various drugs were used. The infection rate was lower in the antibiotic group.[15] Prophylactic antibiotics do not reduce infection rates in most lacerations, but many clinicians recognize that primary puncture wound care is limited and they anticipate the criticism of expert witnesses if infection develops.[16]

If a clinician decides to use prophylactic therapy, particularly for immunocompromised patients, some of the fluoroquinolones may be a good choice.

They currently have acceptable activity against *Pseudomonas aeruginosa*, staphylococci, streptococci, and some clostridial species.[17,18]

DECISION MAKING AND FOLLOW-UP

No scientific evidence favors one management strategy over another for plantar puncture wounds. When the optimal management of a problem in medicine is unknown, it is best to involve the patient in the decision-making process. Because these puncture wounds are so difficult to explore and clean, physicians should re-evaluate them for infection within 2 to 3 days and aggressively search for a retained foreign body if infection develops at any time. **Development of infection in a plantar puncture wound is highly suggestive of a retained foreign body.**

REFERENCES

1. Fitzgerald, RH, and Cowan, JDE: Puncture wounds of the foot. Orthop Clin North Am 6:965–972, 1975.
2. Graham, BS, and Gregory, DW: Pseudomonas aeruginosa causing osteomyelitis after puncture wounds of the foot. South Med J 77:1228–1230, 1984.
3. Rahn, KA, and Jacobson, FS: Pseudomonas osteomyelitis of the metatarsal sesamoid bones. Am J Orthop May:365–367, 1997.
4. Houston, AN, Roy, WA, Faust, RA, et al: Tetanus prophylaxis in the treatment of puncture wounds of patients in the deep south. J Trauma 2:439, 1962.
5. Weber, EJ: Plantar puncture wounds: A survey to determine the incidence of infection. J Accid Emerg Med 13:274–277, 1996.
6. Schwab, RA, and Powers, RD: Conservative therapy of plantar puncture wounds. J Emerg Med 13:291–295, 1995.
7. Inaba, AS, Zukin, DD, and Perro, M: An update on the evaluation and management of plantar puncture wounds and Pseudomonas osteomyelitis. Pediatr Emerg Care 8:38–44, 1992.
8. Riegler, HF, and Routson, GW: Complications of deep puncture wounds of the foot. J Trauma 19:18–22, 1979.
9. Edlich, RF, Rodeheaver, GT, Horowitz, JH, et al: Emergency department management of puncture wounds and needlestick exposure. Emerg Med Clin North Am 4:581–582, 1986.
10. Mahan, KT, and Kalish, SR: Complications following puncture wounds of the foot. J Am Podiatr Assoc 72:497–504, 1982.
11. Chisholm, CD, and Schlesser, JF: Plantar puncture wounds: Controversies and treatment recommendations. Ann Emerg Med 18:1352–1357, 1989.
12. Reinherz, RP, Hong, DT, Tisa, LM, et al: Management of puncture wounds in the foot. J Foot Surg 24:288–292, 1985.
13. Miller, EH, and Semian DW: Gram-negative osteomyelitis following puncture wounds of the foot. J Bone Joint Surg 57(suppl A):535–537, 1975.
14. Joseph, WS, and LeFrock, JL: Infections complicting puncture wounds of the foot. J Foot Surg 26(suppl):30–33, 1987.
15. Pennycook, A, Makower, R, and O'Donnell, AM: Puncture wounds of the foot: Can infective complications be avoided? J Royal Soc Med 87:581–583, 1994.
16. Gonzalez, S: Watch your step: Avoiding lawsuits for management of plantar puncture wound. Emergency Legal Briefings 4, 1993.
17. Raz, R, and Miron, D: Oral ciprofloxacin for treatment of infection following nail puncture wounds of the foot. Clin Infect Dis 21:194, 1995.
18. Ramirez-Ronda, CH, Saavedra, S, and Rivera-Vazquez, CR: Comparative, double blind study of oral ciprofloxacin and intravenous cefotaxime in skin and skin structure infections. Am J Med 82(suppl 4A):220–223, 1987.

CHARLES V. POLLACK, JR., MD

CHAPTER

15

Cutaneous and Subcutaneous Abscesses

Abscesses are surgical lesions. They are localized collections of inflammatory and infectious products completely or nearly completely encapsulated by firm granulation tissue. Abscesses are common problems that account for 1 to 2 percent of all emergency department visits in the United States.[1] The typical cutaneous manifestations of abscesses are erythema, tenderness, and induration with or without fluctuance. Abscesses occur throughout the body, on cutaneous and mucosal surfaces; approximately 20 percent occur on the head and neck, 25 percent in the buttock and perineal area, 25 percent in the axillae, 15 percent in the inguinal area, and 18 percent elsewhere on the extremities.[2] The anatomical location is an efficient determinant for the classification of abscesses, unlike other infectious processes, which are typically classed by microbiologic etiology. Cutaneous abscesses are more common in patients with inflammatory bowel disease and various immune deficiencies such as chronic granulomatous disease and HIV infection; other patients have a tendency to develop recurrent staphylococcal furuncles or infected sebaceous cysts.

In immunocompetent patients, cutaneous and subcutaneous abscesses are typically local phenomena, caused by staphylococcal and streptococcal skin flora, and are not associated with systemic toxicity. Signs of infection beyond local erythema and associated lymphangitis should prompt suspicion of deeper tissue involvement or bacteremia.[3,4] Abscesses in immunocompromised patients should be approached with great respect. Early recognition is essential to effective management, and the nature of the immune deficiency may mask typical cutaneous signs of severity.[4]

The microbiology of abscesses is generally well understood. They originate from a breakdown in the usual epidermal defenses. Therefore, most cutaneous abscesses are caused by skin flora: staphylococci in most areas, and anaerobic bacteria in the perioral (usually gram-positive bacteria) and perianal (usually gram-negative bacteria) regions. Important exceptions to this rule include abscesses resulting from trauma, such as a bite wound, when foreign bacteria are injected under the epidermis. Less commonly, a deep tissue abscess may extend into the skin. Much rarer are hematogenously seeded skin infections such as that classically ascribed to bacterial endocarditis.

Cutaneous abscesses are particularly prone to occur around hair follicles, after abrasions or lacerations, after self-treatment for abrasions (which frequently results in maceration of the skin), and around foreign bodies such as sutures (which allow bacteria to gain ready access to subcutaneous tissues usually protected by intact epidermis).[4,5] Whether or not this microbial penetration results in cellulitis or abscess formation depends on the size of the inoculum, the virulence of the organism, and a variety of host factors. The body's attempt to sequester the infection and resulting inflammation may result in abscess formation.

If one is not sure whether an area of induration and erythema represents an abscess (e.g., when fluctuance is lacking), diagnostic needle aspiration can be considered. If pus is identified, formal incision and drainage (I&D) should then be performed. Ultrasound may also prove to be useful in identifying local collections of pus.

A thorough patient history and physical examination should always precede treatment of all but the most minor and obvious cutaneous abscesses. Issues of interest include any evidence of immune compromise, any systemic symptoms that may give clues to the diagnosis of an underlying disease much more complex than the abscess, and characteristics of the abscess (e.g., the presence of vesicles) that may suggest an alternative diagnosis. These issues are discussed further in this chapter.

TREATMENT

Treatment of cutaneous and subcutaneous abscesses is attended by several significant questions:

1. Can the infection be treated with antimicrobial agents alone or should a drainage procedure be performed?
2. If a drainage procedure is chosen, should antibiotics be given before the procedure in case the procedure itself causes bacteremia?
3. If a drainage procedure is chosen, is needle aspiration sufficient or should formal I&D be performed?
4. If I&D is chosen, how should the procedure be performed?
5. If I&D completely empties the abscess cavity, is subsequent antibiotic therapy indicated?
6. Should immunocompromised patients be managed differently from immunocompetent patients?
7. Are there abscesses or similarly appearing processes that should be managed differently in the emergency department?

THE ROLE OF ANTIBIOTICS

Antibiotics alone are inadequate treatment for a localized collection of pus.[5] The body encapsulates cutaneous and subcutaneous abscesses with dense fibrous tissue in an effort to prevent them from spreading and, in so doing, also effectively reduces the blood supply to the infectious focus. Antibiotics do not concentrate sufficiently in these highly inflamed areas to ensure bactericidal effect.[5]

Sometimes an abscess may not be amenable to drainage on initial presentation. Premature incision into an abscess before it is well localized may actually allow the harmful spread of infection into adjacent and deeper tissues. In these situations, it may be appropriate to treat with antibiotics for 24 to 48 hours while the abscess "ripens," perhaps with the help of hot compresses. Resolution of the lesion during this time implies that the pathologic process was cellulitis and not an abscess, and it should not be construed as supporting nonsurgical management of true cutaneous and subcutaneous abscesses.

In individuals at risk for endocarditis (e.g., immunocompromised patients, patients with artificial heart valves or joints), it is advisable to administer empiric antimicrobial prophylaxis before I&D.[6] Sharp instrumentation of an abscess clearly has the potential to seed the bloodstream with bacteria from the abscess, even in immunocompetent patients.[7] An antistaphylococcal penicillin (dicloxacillin 2 g) or first-generation cephalosporin (cephalexin 2 g) is an appropriate choice to be given orally 1 hour before the procedure. For patients who are allergic to penicillins, clindamycin (600 mg), azithromycin (500 mg), or clarithromycin (500 mg) are acceptable alternatives. For those unable to take oral antibiotics or who are known to have methicillin-resistant *Staphylococcus aureus* bacteremia, vancomycin (1 g) is the regimen of choice.[6] The American Heart Association's recommendations do not expressly apply to patients with noncardiac prostheses such as artificial joints or indwelling intravascular catheters. Directed questioning of patients or the family and careful documentation regarding the patient's risk of endocarditis should always be conducted.

DRAINAGE

Needle Aspiration versus Incision and Drainage

Thorough drainage of an abscess is achieved only by I&D, not by aspiration. The only reasonable indication for needle aspiration of a suspected abscess is for diagnostic confirmation of the presence of pus when fluctuance is lacking or when sterile hematoma or seroma are differential considerations. If pus is found, then formal I&D should follow. Ultrasound can be used to guide needle placement and delineate the extent of the abscess cavity.[8] Incomplete drainage is painful, inefficient, and needlessly prolongs the patient's course of treatment. Abscesses in cosmetically important areas can often be drained from the mucosal side (e.g., a facial abscess may be drained through the buccal mucosa), but even when this is not possible, the inadequacy of needle aspiration still argues against its use.

Performance of Incision and Drainage

Incision and drainage is an exquisitely painful procedure performed in an area already rife with inflammation and pain. After consideration of prophylactic antibiotic coverage, the clinician's next efforts should be directed at adequate anesthesia and analgesia (see Chapters 4 and 5). This is not only a humane approach, but it also facilitates thorough exploration of the abscess cavity and dissection of any septations inside.

Typical infiltrated local anesthetics such as lidocaine are notoriously ineffective in areas of inflammation, increased tissue pressure, and thin skin.[9] Gentle subcutaneous infiltration across the dome of the abscess (Fig. 15–1) anesthetizes the patient to the incision but not to the deeper exploration and dissection. Systemic analgesia or procedural sedation are generally effective for abscess drainage in the emergency department (see Chapter 5). Ethyl chloride spray is a poor choice of anesthetic agent in all but the most superficial of abscesses.

It is generally true that the larger the abscess, the more analgesia is needed, but this is only true up to a practical limit. Larger, more complex abscesses; those in particularly frail, ill, or immunocompromised patients; or those in exquisitely well-innervated areas such as the perineum should be considered for formal surgical I&D in the operating room under the influence of more powerful anesthetic agents. Occasionally, performance of a field block around the abscess will allow a relatively painless I&D procedure (Fig. 15–2).

After anesthesia or analgesia and identification of anatomic structures that may interfere (e.g., superficial blood vessels, nerves, or muscles and tendons), a single stab wound extended into a linear (not cruciate) incision is made across the length of the fluctuant area with a No. 11 scalpel blade (Fig. 15–3). The abscess cavity should be entered with the stab; avoid "sawing" or "probing" to find pus. Whenever possible, the direction of the incision should be parallel to the lines of minimal tension (see Fig. 1–3) to optimize scarring after drainage. **Beware of incision of a pulsatile abscess or one over large blood vessels.** Occasionally ultrasound of the abscess may help distinguish between a true abscess and a pseudoaneurysm, which should never be incised.

Liberated pus can be irrigated or suctioned away. **In immunocompetent patients, Gram stain or culture of abscess contents is rarely clinically useful or cost effective.**[10] In acutely toxic and immunocompromised patients,

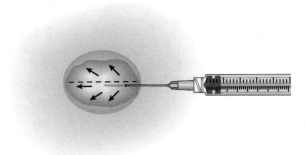

FIG. 15–1. Anesthetizing the incision site. The anesthetic is injected in the subcutaneous plane under the area of the planned incision.

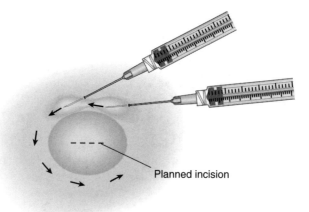

FIG. 15–2. Performing a field block around the abscess. Local anesthetic is injected in a circular fashion around the éntire area of the abscess.

specimens for microbiologic study (including anaerobic cultures) to detect atypical or resistant pathogens are best obtained by sterile needle aspiration before I&D is done.[10]

After the cavity is opened, it is essential that it is thoroughly and systematically explored. This should be done bluntly, with a hemostat or (size allowing)

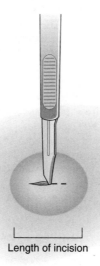

FIG. 15–3. Method of incision of an abscess using a No. 11 surgical blade. The area of maximal fluctuance is incised with a gentle stabbing motion with the tip of the blade.

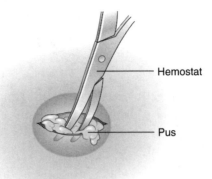

FIG. 15–4. After incising the abscess, the cavity is explored with a curved hemostat. The hemostat is inserted into all recesses of the abscess. By repeatedly spreading its jaws, any fibrous septations are broken down.

a gloved finger. This is the most painful portion of the procedure for the patient (Fig. 15–4). Additional local anesthesia is often required. Through the years, various authors have recommended irrigating the cavity out with saline, dilute hydrogen peroxide, or dilute betadine, but none of these has been associated with a change in outcome.

The incision should not be closed, even in cosmetic areas. The cavity should be packed with ribbon gauze. **The incision into a deep or expansive cutaneous abscess should be kept open with a wick after the procedure, but it is not necessary to fully "pack" the abscess cavity.** Although all nooks and crannies of the cavity should be drained and then packed, the wound should not be packed tightly because this practice traps purulence in the cavity and may enlarge the eventual scar. The goal is to apply the packing gauze to all surfaces of the cavity so that its surface is gently débrided when the gauze is removed. Packing generally promotes hemostasis, but abscess I&D is not typically a bloody procedure. (In extremity abscesses, a tourniquet can be placed before I&D is done.)

The gauze should be removed in 48 hours. This should be done in a prearranged wound check examination scheduled at the time of the I&D procedure. If purulent drainage persists, the cavity should be re-explored, irrigated, and repacked. After the gauze removed is dry and clean, further packing is of no benefit.

POSTPROCEDURE ANTIBIOTIC TREATMENT

Thorough drainage of an abscess often obviates the need for antibiotic therapy. For the vast majority of otherwise healthy patients, antibiotics have no proven benefit after successful I&D.[1,11] High-risk patients have not been studied in this regard, but there are suggestions scattered throughout the literature[9] indicating postsurgical antibiotic therapy for patients with the following conditions:

- Immune compromise
- Systemic toxicity (e.g., fever, chills, rigors)
- Recurrent abscesses
- Significant surrounding cellulitis or proximal lymphangitis
- Abscesses in high-risk areas (e.g., the central face)
- Any condition for which preprocedure antibiotics are deemed appropriate, even if the drainage is apparently successful.

Inadequate drainage *per se* is *not* an indication for antibiotics; rather, it is an indication for better drainage, in the operating room if necessary. As already discussed, the choice of antibiotics is best guided by the location of the abscess.

IMMUNOCOMPROMISED PATIENTS

Much anecdotal experience and excruciatingly few good data support the use of empiric antibiotic therapy as an adjunct to I&D for treatment of abscesses in immunocompromised patients. A broad definition of "immunocompromise" is appropriate in this regard, and includes patients with HIV and AIDS; diabetes; chronic use of corticosteroids; organ transplant patients taking immunosuppressants; patients receiving chemotherapy for malignancy; alcoholics; malnourished patients; and even patients with significant liver, heart, or lung disease, whose overall humoral immunity might be questionable.

As already mentioned, for immunocompromised patients, it might be worthwhile to perform Gram stain and culture of the abscess contents, both to direct empiric therapy and to provide good alternative choices if initial treatment fails. Antibiotics should be given until the infection resolves.

DIFFERENTIAL DIAGNOSIS, DIFFERENTIAL MANAGEMENT, AND SPECIAL CONSIDERATIONS

Special considerations in the emergency department care of cutaneous and subcutaneous abscesses include specific predilections for nonstaphylococcal, nonstreptococcal etiologies, and some skin lesions that may appear to be simple cutaneous abscesses but actually are not. **Apparent abscesses that must be approached with great caution include those overlying the frontal bone and sinus, the chest wall, and the peritoneal cavity. Patients with some systemic diseases, such as malignancies or sarcoidosis, should also be carefully evaluated before drainage of an apparent cutaneous abscess is attempted.**

- *Folliculitis, furuncles, and carbuncles.* Folliculitis is a very common skin infection, almost always caused by *Staphylococcus aureus*. Abscesses originate around hair follicles, but after they are established, they may either "point" externally or may track more deeply, which is a common cause of bacterial endocarditis.[9] Simple folliculitis typically responds to local cleansing and wound care. More extensive staphylococcal abscesses are referred to as *boils* or *furuncles*, and clusters of furuncles are termed *carbuncles*. Furuncles are treated with I&D in a conventional fashion; carbuncles frequently require formal surgical drainage in the operating room.

- *Hidradenitis suppurativa.* Hidradenitis is a chronic inflammatory condition of the apocrine glands in the axilla and groin. Secondary infection typically results in extensive abscess formation and fistulization. Recurrent I&Ds cause significant scarring, and wider drainage procedures are eventually indicated. Although anaerobic bacteria are frequently isolated from hidradenitis suppurativa, staphylococci remain the most common cause of infection. After the condition is no longer amenable to routine I&D, patients should receive antibiotic therapy pending surgical evaluation.

- *Pilonidal cyst abscesses.* Pilonidal sinuses, cysts, and abscesses are relatively common findings in the sacrococcygeal region. Pilonidal sinuses are congenital lesions, but they are not usually evident until adolescence, when body hair starts to increase. Drainage of a pilonidal abscess should always include a search for and removal of hair and follicular tissue at the base of the cavity. Because of the possibility of fecal soilage, these lesions may require broad-spectrum antibiotic coverage. Simple I&D temporarily relieves symptoms, but formal excision of the cyst cavity is often required to prevent recurrence.

- *Breast abscesses.* Although mastitis and breast abscess during breastfeeding are common, nonpuerperal mastitis is actually more frequently encountered. All these are typically managed with routine I&D, but periareolar abscesses are more problematic because they tend to be polymicrobial and because fluctuance may be deep and difficult to appreciate. Deeper breast abscesses typically require formal surgical drainage.[12] If the infection does not resolve within several days, inflammatory breast cancer should be considered.

- *Bartholin's gland abscesses.* Bartholin's gland abscess management differs in two ways from the management of other cutaneous and subcutaneous processes: first, it is expected that gram-negative organisms, particularly gonococci and coliforms, will predominate as infectious agents. Cervical cultures should be taken for gonorrhea when the abscess is treated. Second, a specific device, the Word catheter, is used in the drainage of the abscesses; it allows complete drainage and subsequent iatrogenic fistulization of the abscess (Fig. 15–5). The incision, through the mucosal surface of the labia, should be made only large enough to admit the uninflated catheter tip, and the balloon should be filled with a sufficient volume of water to prevent extrusion without causing persistent pain. Before insertion of the catheter, all purulent material should be drained. The Word catheter is intended to be left in place for 6 to 8 weeks to allow fistulization to occur and prevent recurrence.[13] Persistent infection, especially in older patients, should raise the possibility of an inflammatory cancer.

- *Lymphogranuloma venereum* (LGV). LGV is a sexually transmitted disease caused by *Chlamydia trachomatis.* It typically manifests as unilateral, painful, swollen, suppurative inguinal or femoral lymph nodes. Although these lesions may

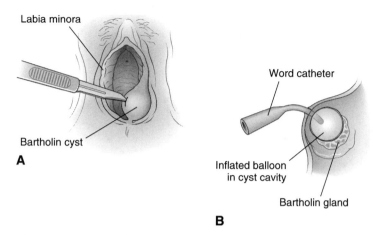

Labia minora

Word catheter

Bartholin cyst

A

Inflated balloon
in cyst cavity

Bartholin gland

B

FIG. 15–5. The Word catheter. *(A)* A small incision is made on the mucosal side of the labia over the area of maximal fluctuance. *(B)* After drainage of any purulent material, the end of the catheter is inserted through the incision and the bulb is inflated with 2 to 3 mL of normal saline.

look like abscesses, they should not be drained because fistulization is a likely undesirable sequela. Serology is more accurate in making the diagnosis than aspiration and culture, which is notoriously unreliable. The preferred treatment is oral doxycycline 100 mg bid (twice a day) for 21 days.[14]

- *Paronychia.* Paronychia is an infection of the potential space between the nail cuticle and the nail root. It typically occurs around the fingernails but may also affect toenails. Paronychia is usually a staphylococcal infection, but anaerobes may be found, particularly in patients who suck their fingers or bite their fingernails. The usual progression of illness is hangnail to cellulitis to abscess. Adequate I&D of paronychia does not typically require removal of the nail. Anesthesia may be necessary and is best effected by a digital approach. These lesions are most readily drained by inserting a no. 11 blade scalpel just under the eponychium, parallel to the nail (Fig. 15–6). A small ribbon gauze wick may be used to keep the wound open for 1 to 2 days. Persistence of symptoms for weeks should prompt investigation for osteomyelitis of the distal phalanx.[15]
- *Felon.* Felons are infections of the pulp space of the fingertip. They often result from trauma with or without a retained foreign body, but sometimes the patient cannot identify a specific traumatic cause. Felons are notoriously difficult to drain because of limiting fibrous septations and because of the potential for adverse functional and cosmetic sequelae with improper surgical approach. Drainage through a lateral incision is preferred (Fig. 15–7). The incision should be performed just lateral to the nailfold, and the fibrous septa should be broken down, keeping the exploration dorsal to the neurovascular bundle. Antibiotic coverage (e.g., cephalexin or dicloxacillin) is usually recommended.[9]

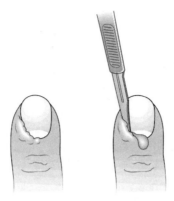

Drainage of paronychia

FIG. 15–6. Drainage of a paronychia with a No. 11 blade. After adequate anesthesia of the digit, the tip of the blade is inserted between the nail and the eponychial fold to drain any purulent material. The incision may be extended by gently sweeping the blade on either side of the original incision.

- *Whitlow.* Herpetic whitlow is a viral infection of the distal phalanx that is caused by *Herpes simplex*. At some point in their natural history, these infections manifest typical herpetic vesicles. However, on emergency department presentation, these are not always evident, and the fingertip may appear to be abscessed. Obtaining a detailed history for the presence of vesicles is important because whitlow does not respond to I&D. In fact, it may worsen after I&D owing to bacterial superinfection.[16]
- *Pott's puffy tumor.* Pott's puffy tumor is a subperiosteal abscess of the frontal bone that occurs as a complication of frontal sinusitis. Classically, this le-

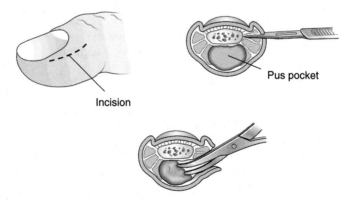

Incision

Pus pocket

FIG. 15–7. Lateral technique for drainage of a felon. The No. 11 blade is inserted through the lateral aspect of the fingertip, avoiding contact with the digital vessels. After drainage of any purulent material, the tip of a curved hemostat is inserted into the abscess cavity to break down the fibrous septations.

sion is manifested as an indolent, puffy, circumscribed swelling of the forehead. Fully developed, Pott's puffy tumor has the appearance of an abscess
of the forehead. It is increasingly rare in this era of broad-spectrum antibiotics. Surgical drainage is the treatment of choice, but it should not be performed without a preceding computed tomography (CT) scan of the head to
determine the extent of frontal bone involvement. These infections tend to
be polymicrobial, and antibiotic therapy is guided by culture results.[17]

- *Granulomata.* A number of granulomatous syndromes may manifest skin lesions that appear to be cutaneous or subcutaneous abscesses. Wegener's
granulomatosis may present with perirectal or perianal lesions, and sarcoidosis may cause erythema nodosum and other skin lesions that may be
mistaken for routine abscesses.[18] Careful attention should be paid to obtaining a thorough history in patients with abscess and any other skin lesions, otherwise unexplained pulmonary or gastrointestinal symptoms, or
systemic symptoms consistent with chronic disease.
- *Skin lesions of Crohn's disease.* Likewise, Crohn's disease is sometimes accompanied by skin lesions, which may variably appear as nodules, abscesses, or
ulcers. These are not known to precede the gastrointestinal symptoms.
These lesions may become secondarily infected but otherwise routinely respond to anti-inflammatory medications.[19]
- *Neoplastic extension.* There are occasional case reports[20] of internal malignancies presenting as cutaneous abscesses. Biopsy of the abscess wall may reveal the underlying diagnosis, but it is not likely to be performed in the
emergency department or the primary care setting. Again, this unusual relationship reinforces the value of a thorough patient history and physical examination in patients with cutaneous and subcutaneous abscesses.
- *Deep abscess extension.* Likewise, untreated deep abscesses may manifest cuta-
neously. This should be suspected particularly in patients with diabetes or
other immunocompromising conditions. When abscesses occur on the abdominal wall or chest wall, CT scanning should be considered before I&D is
attempted and the deep tissues are inadvertently exposed.[21]
- *Vibrio infections.* Although classically presenting as skin necrosis with bullous
lesions, skin infections with *Vibrio vulnificus* may present early as abscesses.
These patients tend to be rather ill, and their prognosis without aggressive
surgical treatment is poor. A history of any exposure of a wound to salt water or any recent ingestion of raw shellfish should be sought. Patients with
liver disease and infection caused by *Vibrio* organisms may have particularly
rapid downhill courses.[22]
- *Necrotizing soft tissue infections.* Necrotizing soft tissue infections (e.g., pannic-
ulitis, necrotizing fasciitis, myositis, osteomyelitis) may present early with
simple cutaneous abscess. This may be more likely in injection drug users.[3]
These illnesses can be detected early only with a thorough history and physical examination and close follow-up.
- *Furuncular myiasis.* Furuncular myiasis is caused by invasion of viable skin by
the larval maggots of various species of flies. These lesions are most often
seen in natives of or recent visitors to Africa or Central or South America.
Unlike abscesses, myiasis lesions have a central opening through which the
maggot breathes. In addition, the patient experiences lancinating pain when
the maggot moves. The most atraumatic treatment for such lesions is to

suffocate the maggot by covering the breathing opening for several hours. When the maggot tries to come out for air, it can be extruded by firm lateral pressure on the lesion.[23] Larvae are sometimes discovered unexpectedly upon routine abscess I&D.[24] A history of travel is necessary to make the diagnosis before intervening.

REFERENCES

1. Llera, JL, and Levy, RC: Treatment of cutaneous abscess: A double-blind clinical study. Ann Emerg Med 14:15–19, 1985.
2. Peter, G, and Smith, AL: Group A streptococci infections of the skin and pharynx. N Engl J Med 297:311–317, 1977.
3. Callahan, TE, Schecter, WP, and Horn, JK: Necrotizing soft tissue infection masquerading as cutaneous abscess following illicit drug injection. Arch Surg 133:812–818, 1998.
4. Bisno, AL, and Stevens, DL: Streptococcal infections of skin and soft tissues. N Engl J Med 334:240–245, 1996.
5. Llera, JL, Levy, RC, and Staneck, JL: Cutaneous abscesses: Natural history and management in an outpatient facility. J Emerg Med 1:489–493, 1984.
6. Dijani, AS, Taubert, KA, Wilson, W, et al: Prevention of bacterial endocarditis. Recommendations by the American Heart Association. JAMA 277:1794–1801, 1997.
7. Le Frock, JL, and Molavi, A: Transient bacteremia associated with diagnostic and therapeutic procedures. Comp Ther 8:65–71, 1982.
8. Baurmash, HD: Ultrasonography in the diagnosis and treatment of facial abscess. J Oral Maxillofac Surg 57:635–636, 1999.
9. Stapczynski, JS: Skin and Soft-Tissue Infections. In Brillman, JC, and Quenzer, RW (eds): Infectious Disease in Emergency Medicine, ed. 2. Lippincott-Raven, Philadelphia, 1998, pp 755–790.
10. Meislin, HW: Management and microbiology of cutaneous abscesses. JACEP 7:186–191, 1978.
11. Blick, PWH, Flowers, MW, Marsden, AK, et al: Antibiotics in surgical treatment of acute abscesses. Br J Med 281:111–112, 1980.
12. Watt-Boolsen, S, Rasmussen, NR, and Blichert-Toft, M: Primary periareolar abscess in the non-lactating breast: Risk of recurrence. Am J Surg 153:571–573, 1987.
13. Word, B: Office treatment of cyst and abscess of Bartholin's gland duct. South Med J 61:514–518, 1968.
14. Rosen, T, and Brown, TJ: Cutaneous manifestations of sexually transmitted diseases. Med Clin N Am 82:1081–1104, 1998.
15. Zook, EG, and Brown, RE: The perinychium. In Green, DP, Hotchkiss, RN, and Pederson, WC (eds): Operative Hand Surgery, ed. 4. Churchill Livingstone, New York, 1999, pp 1353–1380.
16. Feder, HM, and Long, SS: Herpetic whitlow: Epidemiology, clinical characteristics, diagnosis, and treatment. Am J Dis Child 137:861–863, 1983.
17. Babu, RP: Pott's puffy tumor: The forgotten entity. J Neurosurg 84:110–112, 1996.
18. Mañá, J, Marcoval, J, Graells, J, et al: Cutaneous involvement in sarcoidosis. Arch Dermatol 133:882–888, 1997.
19. Hackzell-Bradley, M, Hedblad, M-A, and Stephansson, EA: Metastatic Crohn's disease: report of 3 cases with special reference to histopathologic findings. Arch Dermatol 132:928–932, 1996.
20. Mann, GN, Scroggins, CR, and Adkins, B: Perforated cecal adenocarcinoma presenting as a thigh abscess. South Med J 90:949–951, 1997.
21. Bobrow, BJ, Mohr, J, and Pollack, CV Jr: An unusual complication of missed appendicitis. J Emerg Med 14:719–722, 1996.
22. Pollack, CV Jr, and Fuller, J: Update on emerging infections: Outbreak of Vibrio parahaemolyticus infection associated with eating raw oysters and clams harvested from Long Island Sound. Ann Emerg Med 34:679–680, 1999.
23. Kain, KC: Skin lesions in the returned traveler. Med Clin N Am 83:1077–1102, 1999.
24. Johnston, M, and Dickinson, G: An unexpected surprise in a common boil. J Emerg Med 14:779–781, 1996.

HARRY S. SOROFF, MD
J.J. CRUZ, MD
JOHN S. BREBBIA, MD

CHAPTER

16

Burns

Each year, between 1 and 2 million burns are sustained in the United States alone.[1] Fortunately, most of the burns are small, and the care of victims focuses on local wound care.[2] Initial care of burn victims should address life-threatening injuries that compromise vital functions, including the airway, breathing, and circulation. For optimal follow-up, one should refer all but the most minor burns to a burn center if one is available. **The response to burns is determined by the total area of the body surface burned and the depth of the burns.** Accurate assessments of burn extent and depth are required to determine the appropriate therapy for the burn injury. Avoiding infection and further damage to the injured tissues will help optimize healing and result in the most aesthetically pleasing and functional scar.

GENERAL PRINCIPLES OF CARE

IMMEDIATE EVALUATION

Before caring for a burn injury, it is important to identify and treat any associated injuries; some burn victims may have other life- or limb-threatening injuries. The immediate evaluation of a patient who has sustained a burn injury includes the following (see later in the chapter for full explanation of some terms):

1. Was the patient burned in an open space or in an enclosed space such as a house? If burns are sustained in a closed space, determine the carboxyhemoglobin level.
2. Is there evidence of smoke inhalation, and is the airway clear?
3. What was the causative agent of the burn (e.g., water, oil, kerosene, gasoline, or an explosive gas such as propane), and is there any evidence of an electrical or chemical injury?

4. What is the extent of the burn, expressed as percentage of the body surface area (BSA)?
5. How much of the body surface has sustained a partial-thickness injury, either superficial or deep, and how much has sustained a full-thickness injury?

PRECAUTIONARY MEASURES

Precautionary ancillary measures in the care of moderate and major burns (all second-degree burns over 15 percent in adults and over 10 percent in children) include:

- A nasogastric tube to prevent gastric ileus and to decompress the stomach from swallowed air
- Intravenous (IV) analgesics (e.g., morphine sulfate) as needed for pain
- Tetanus prophylaxis (tetanus toxoid 0.5 mL). If the immunization history is not known or more than 10 years have elapsed since the last booster, tetanus immunoglobulin (250 U) is also given.

THE EFFECTS OF PATIENT AGE ON BURN MORBIDITY AND MORTALITY

As with other forms of injury, the very young and the elderly experience a higher morbidity and mortality rate from burns. When burns occur in children who are less than 24 months of age, the possibility of either neglect or abuse should always be considered. **Burns in which there is a sharp line of demarcation between the burned and the unburned area suggest immersion, which is suspicious for neglect or abuse.**

Patients older than age 60 years are at high risk, even with a moderate burn, and should be admitted to the hospital. This is especially true for patients with pre-existing diseases such as diabetes mellitus, strokes, or cardiac or respiratory insufficiency. The burn wound itself presents special problems because the thickness of the skin decreases with age. This makes the diagnosis of the depth of the burn more difficult. In elderly patients, one should assume that the burn is deep.

TRANSFER TO A BURN CENTER

Criteria for transfer to a burn center are:

- Third-degree burns over 5 percent of the BSA
- Second- or third-degree burns over 15 percent of the BSA (10% in children younger than age 10 years)
- Electrical burns

- Inhalation injury
- Patient is elderly (age > 60 years) or has severe comorbidity
- Burns involve the face, hands, feet, joints, or genitalia

PHYSIOLOGIC ALTERATIONS AFTER BURNS

EARLY CHANGES

Burns are caused by the conduction of thermal energy to the skin from a hot substance such as water, oil, or burning clothing. The effect on the skin depends on both the temperature to which the skin is heated and the time period during which the hot substance is in contact with the skin. Moritz and Henriquez[3] studied these effects in pigs. The early changes, at temperatures between 40 and 44°C, are denaturation of protein and interference with the function of cellular enzyme systems. The sodium pump is one of the most important functions of the cellular membrane that is adversely affected, allowing a high intracellular sodium concentration to develop, which leads to intracellular swelling. Oxygen free radicals are also produced and further aggravate the abnormalities of cell membrane function.[4] As the injury progresses, the cellular proteins become severely altered and eventually progress to cell death or necrosis.

The burn injury is not limited to the surface of the skin; penetration of the heat produces a three-dimensional injury.[4] At the skin surface, there is cell destruction and necrosis. This area is called the *zone of coagulation*. Clinically, this is manifested by the eschar of the full-thickness injury. Beneath the zone of coagulation is a zone of stasis where the cells are initially viable. As the circulation to the area becomes progressively diminished, however, the early ischemia within the zone of stasis may progress to necrosis and the death of cells that were previously viable. With optimal therapy, the circulation improves in the entire zone of stasis, and recovery can occur in 7 to 14 days. During this recovery period, the tissues are very susceptible to injury and infection, however, and must be protected. There is a third, outer zone of hyperemia surrounding the ischemic zone of stasis. In this outer zone, there is minimal cell destruction, and the tissues receive an increase in blood flow, secondary to regional vasodilatation.

FORMATION OF EDEMA

Injury to the capillaries in the burned area impairs their integrity, thus permitting proteins to escape from the serum into the wound.[5] The increased permeability is aggravated by the release of a large number of inflammatory mediators. Even though the edema is most marked in the area of contact with heat, it extends far into the surrounding tissues and interferes with the delivery of oxygen and other nutrients to the injured area, thus aggravating the effect of the ischemia. However, the capillaries retain a selective permeability that keeps large molecules such as fibrinogen and globulin within the vessel while allowing smaller molecules such as albumin to escape into the edema fluid.

The formation of edema begins rapidly, within the first 2 to 3 hours after injury. It then increases, reaches its maximum at about 12 to 24 hours, and persists until 48 to 72 hours. Thereafter, recovery begins with a slow reabsorption that usually takes as long as 7 to 10 days to be completed. The amount of the edema and its duration depend on the severity of the injury. In an extensive or deep burn, the edema becomes massive and continues for a longer period. Fluid therapy (discussed later) is required to prevent the resulting decrease in vascular and intracellular volume from impairing organ function. **The suggested formulas for replacing the intravascular volume lost into the burn edema are largely based on the weight of the patient and the extent of the burn, as expressed in the percentage of BSA involved.**

DETERMINATION OF THE EXTENT OF THE BURN

The extent and the depth of the burn set the stage for the physiologic, metabolic, and anatomic changes that ensue, and they are the major determinants of the chances for the patient's survival. **The percentage of BSA that is burned can be roughly estimated in an adult by the "rule of nines,"[6] in which the head and each upper extremity each comprise 9 percent of the body surface, each lower extremity and the anterior and posterior trunk each comprise 18 percent, and the genitalia comprise 1 percent** (Fig. 16–1). A good

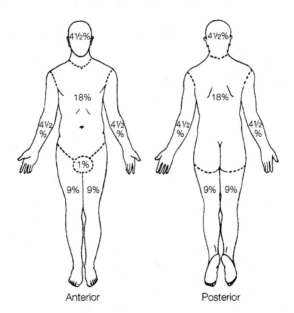

Anterior   Posterior

FIG. 16–1. Estimating the percent of total body surface area of burns in adults. (From Lund, CC, and Browder, NE: The estimation of areas of burns. Surgery, Gynecology and Obstetrics 79:357, 1944. As adapted by: Clayton, MC and Solem, LD: No ice, no butter. Advice on management of burns for primary care physicians. Postgrad Med 97:151–165, 1995, with permission.)

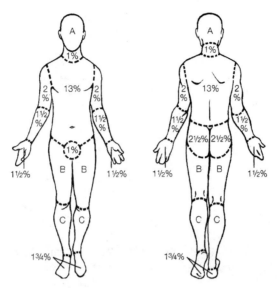

Relative percentages of areas affected by growth

Age	Half of head (A)	Half of one thigh (B)	Half of one leg (C)
Infant	9½	2¾	2½
1 yr	8½	3¼	2½
5 yr	6½	4	2¾
10 yr	5½	4¼	3
15 yr	4½	4½	3¼
Adult	3½	4¾	3½

FIG. 16–2. Estimating the percent of total body surface area of burns in children. (From Lund CC, and Browder NE: The estimation of areas of burns. Surgery, Gynecology and Obstetrics 79:357, 1944. As adapted by: Clayton MC and Solem LD: No ice, no butter. Advice on management of burns for primary care physicians. Postgrad Med 1995;97:151–165, with permission.)

estimate can be made by using the chart developed by Lund and Browder,[7] which takes into account the differences in relative surface areas of the body that exist in infants and how they change with growth (Fig. 16–2). **In adults, the area of the palm of the hand is equivalent to approximately 1 percent of the BSA.**

DETERMINATION OF BURN DEPTH

Burns are usually classified either as partial- or full-thickness burns based on the degree of damage to the dermis. Partial-thickness burns may be either superficial or deep. Full-thickness burns may also extend deeper into the fascia and muscle.

Superficial (first-degree) burns are most commonly caused by the ultraviolet rays of the sun. It may also be caused by a brief exposure to heat, such as occurs in an explosion of propane gas. **Even though first-degree burns are painful and may be associated with minimal edema, they almost always heal in 3 to 5 days.**

Superficial partial-thickness (second-degree) burns are characterized by the presence of blisters and a weeping, erythematous skin surface. Because the nerve endings are intact, this type of burn is associated with a great deal of pain. Burns of this depth, which can result from hot oil used for cooking or from extended exposure to hot water or steam, are very common. Patients with superficial second-degree burns should be followed carefully. The burned area should be checked frequently to determine whether the depth of the injury is progressing. The injured surface contains many viable exposed nerve endings, so dressing changes are extremely painful despite the use of analgesics.

Probably the most difficult burns to diagnose are *deep partial-thickness* or *deep dermal burns*. The wound should be observed and dressed daily in order to determine whether the depth becomes more severe with the passage of time. **Deep dermal burns that do not heal in 21 days should probably be excised and grafted because scarring is common when healing does occur.** The surface of the deep dermal burn is formed by injured collagen, which is light tan or white and adheres to the deeper tissues. Over a period of days, as the dead and denatured collagen of the injured dermis is gradually débrided, it exposes a normal hyperemic layer of dermis, which contains numerous epithelial papillae or islands from which new epithelium grows to resurface and heal the burned area. This new epithelium is friable and liable to injury for some time.

The diagnosis of *full-thickness* or *third-degree burns* is usually obvious on presentation. The burned surface is dry and leathery in texture and is insensate. There are no viable hairs in the injured area. If the destruction is severe, the area may actually be charred, with thrombosed vessels visible within the eschar. It is more difficult, however, to diagnose a full-thickness injury that evolves over time from a deep dermal injury. This diagnosis may be complicated if the amount of heat applied to different portions of the body is not uniform; in such cases, an area of deep dermal injury that will heal may be next to an area of full-thickness burn that requires excision and grafting.

Deeper burns can involve muscle, fascia, nerves, and even bone. The most common causes of such a devastating injury is the passage of high-voltage electricity through the body or the prolonged exposure of portions of the body to heat of a high intensity, which can occur when gasoline ignites clothing or the person is trapped in a closed space.

FLUID THERAPY

The rationale for providing fluid therapy is to replace the intravascular and intracellular fluid that is lost into the burn wound in the form of edema. If this intravascular fluid is not replaced, then the resulting decrease in vascular and intracellular volume after a large burn will cause impaired organ function and ultimately death.

Lactated Ringer's solution is the most commonly used form of fluid replacement. It has a sodium content of 130 mEq/L, and its composition approximates that of the extracellular fluid that is lost into the edema. **The most popular formula for fluid administration is the Parkland formula (4 mL × body weight in kilograms × percentage of the BSA burned).** Because the burn wound edema forms most rapidly in the first 8 hours after injury, it has been recommended that half of the first day's fluid budget be administered during this period, and the third and fourth quarters should be given during each of the ensuing 8-hour periods. The adequacy of the fluid replacement can be gauged from the volume of urine output. In an adult, if the hourly urine output is 30 to 50 mL/h (or about 0.5 mL/kg body weight in children), it is presumed that the fluid volume replacement is adequate. If the urine output falls to 10 to 15 mL/h, the rate of fluid administration should be accelerated. A urine output that exceeds 60 mL/h suggests that the rate of fluid administration should be adjusted downward.

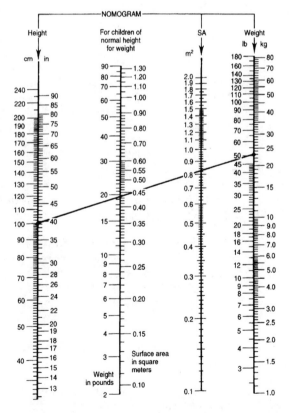

FIG. 16–3. Nomogram for determining surface area based on height and weight in children. (From Herndon, DN, Rutan, RL, Alison, WE, Jr, and Cox, CS, Jr: Management of burn injuries. In Eichelberger, MR (ed): Pediatric Trauma: Prevention, Acute Care, Rehabilitation. St. Louis, Mosby Year Book, 1993, p. 572, with permission.)

In children, the surface areas of the various parts of the body are different from those of adults. For example, children's heads represent a larger percentage of their surface area than do their limbs. The relationship between surface area and weight in adults does not pertain to growing children. The fluid requirements for resuscitation of children should be based on surface area, which can be determined from a nomogram such as that shown in Figure 16–3. During the first 24 hours, the volume of lactated Ringer's solution should be 5000 mL per square meter of body surface burn. Children should also be given 2000 mL of 5% glucose in water per square meter of body surface to make up for insensible losses.

A patient who has suffered a crush or electrical injury may produce dark red urine owing to myoglobin or hemoglobin. Sodium bicarbonate should be added to the IV fluids to alkalinize the urine.

INHALATION INJURY

It has been estimated that about 20 to 30 percent of patients exposed to fires experience an element of smoke inhalation injury and carbon monoxide intoxication. The possibility of such an inhalation injury must be evaluated in every burn patient because it is one of the major determinants of morbidity and mortality. Fire and the combustion products of a wide variety of materials create heated gases containing particulate matter as smoke. The history of where the fire occurred is important because the smoke and heated gases are the most concentrated when they are in a closed space. Direct heat is injurious to the upper airway; it initiates the formation of edema, which obstructs the free movement of air. For this reason, it is recommended that all burn victims should receive humidified oxygen at a concentration of 100 percent at the scene of the fire.[8]

The symptoms that should alert the clinician to inhalation injury are hoarseness, stridor, a severe barking cough, and wheezing. **The presence of carbonaceous material in and around the mouth and singed nasal hairs are clear evidence that smoke inhalation has occurred.** In addition to examining the status of the airway, the expansion of the patient's chest should also be observed. **If there are full-thickness circumferential burns of the chest, which will compromise respiratory excursions, emergent escharotomies should be planned.** In the presence of a face or neck burn and evidence of smoke inhalation, endotracheal intubation should be considered. This should be carried out in the emergency room before the development of edema makes it difficult. It is preferable to insert an endotracheal tube of adequate caliber to enable frequent lavage, suctioning, and bronchoscopy. After the patient has been stabilized, fiberoptic bronchoscopy should be performed, and it should be repeated until the inhaled particles of soot are removed.

In young children, the small caliber of the airway makes them especially vulnerable to narrowing caused by edema; even a small decrease in the cross-sectional area of the airway can cause a significant increase in airway resistance. Direct laryngoscopy and bronchoscopy allow the clinician to determine whether soot is present in the trachea and permit lavage and the concurrent placement of an endotracheal tube. If these measures cannot be performed because of severe edema, then an emergent cricothyroidotomy or tracheostomy should be carried out.

When patients are burned in a closed space, the air may be deficient in oxygen and contain carbon monoxide. Carbon monoxide in the blood shifts the oxygen dissociation curve to the left, which inhibits the release of oxygen to the tissues. The patient may then develop neurologic or cardiac abnormalities. A carboxyhemoglobin concentration of greater than 15 percent is toxic, and one greater than 50 percent can be lethal. The patient may exhibit symptoms of headache, irritability, visual disturbances, and impaired judgment.[9] The treatment for carbon monoxide toxicity is delivery of a high concentration of oxygen. Patients with severe exposures are administered 100 percent oxygen in a hyperbaric chamber at 2.5 atmospheres for 30 minutes. More than one session may be required.

When polymers containing nitrogen are burned, they may produce hydrogen cyanide. The presence of hydrogen cyanide should be suspected in patients in whom an odor of bitter almonds is detected. The symptoms include lethargy, nausea, and headache, and may progress to coma. The treatment includes IV sodium thiosulfate 125 to 250 mg/kg and hydroxycobalamin 4 g, as well as 100 percent oxygen.

LOCAL CARE OF THE BURN WOUND

FIRST-DEGREE BURNS

Patients with first-degree burns require only symptomatic care. Patients are more comfortable if the burn is covered with an ointment such as petrolatum or aloe vera or an ointment containing an analgesic, in order to relieve the local pain caused by the movement of air over the wound. There is no need for topical antibiotics. Bed rest and analgesics are recommended for 24 to 48 hours, depending on the extent of the burn. This type of injury resolves itself in that period.

SUPERFICIAL PARTIAL-THICKNESS BURNS (SECOND-DEGREE BURNS)

The most striking manifestation of a superficial second-degree burn is the formation of blisters. The blister is formed by the leakage of serum into the stratum spinosum layer of the epidermis. Plasma proteins and other products of the injured skin are contained within the blister fluid, and these draw more serum into the blister, so that it increases in size over the first 24 hours and sometimes breaks. **The presence of blisters usually indicates that the burn is fairly superficial and that it will heal spontaneously by re-epithelization within 10 days to 2 weeks, providing that no infection occurs.**

Management

After the blisters break, the desquamated skin dries and can be cut away, uncovering the new epithelium that has grown over the surface of the burned area. Studies[10,11] in human volunteers and animals suggest that leaving the burn blisters intact results in more rapid re-epithelization than when the blisters are débrided. **Most blisters should be left intact to allow the outer layer of the blister to function as a biologic dressing.** Large or tense blisters may be aspirated using sterile technique, however, to facilitate their care.

The burned surface can be managed in one of several ways. **The burn can be gently washed with soap and water, and then a topical antimicrobial agent can be applied to the surface.** The most commonly used topical treatment is 1% silver sulfadiazine, which is washed off and replaced twice daily. Bacitracin is also used in superficial burns and on the face. The ear lobes and the nose are especially vulnerable to infection because the skin overlying the poorly vascularized cartilage of these structures is thin. Mafenide acetate (Sulfamylon) should be applied topically, twice daily, to the ear lobes and the tip of the nose. Use of this agent should be limited to small areas, however, because patients often complain of local pain. This agent is also a carbonic anhydrase inhibitor, so if it is used on large burns for long periods, hyperchloremic metabolic acidosis can occur. Its spectrum of activity is against most gram-negative pathogens and most gram-positive bacteria. **Sulfamylon also has an excellent capacity for penetrating the eschar of a full-thickness burn.**

Silver sulfadiazine as a 1% cream is painless and has an *in vitro* activity against a wide range of organisms, including S. *aureus*, E. *coli*, *Klebsiella* spp., *Pseudomonas aeruginosa*, *Enterobacter* spp., and *Proteus* spp.. The most common toxic side effect of this agent is a transient leukopenia, which can manifest itself after several days of therapy as a marked decrease in the neutrophils. The leukopenia tends to go away after the use of the cream is stopped. A small number of patients experience a maculopapular rash, which also disappears after the sulfadiazine is stopped.

Alternative Burn Dressings for Superficial Partial-thickness Burns

In the past several decades, a number of synthetic wound coverings have become available. The theory behind the use of such materials is that they do not have to be changed several times daily, they protect the wound, and they decrease the local pain. Epithelization can then proceed under the moist environment of the synthetic dressing and heal the partial-thickness wound. Indeed, a moist environment has been shown to enhance re-epithelization.[12] Biobrane (Bertek Pharmaceuticals, Morgantown, W.Va.) was one of the earliest of these dressings. It is a fabric made up of an inner layer of knitted nylon fibers coated with collagen and an outer layer of silicone. Opsite (Smith & Nephew, Hull, UK) and Tegaderm (3M, St. Paul, Minn.) are transparent films of polyurethane that have adhesive coatings. After the wound is cleaned, these synthetic dressings are applied and fitted snugly to the surface of the wound. If necessary, they can be held in place using an outer layer such as Flexinet (Derma Sciences, Inc., Princeton, N.J.). The wound is then inspected daily; if fluid collects, it can be aspirated using a needle. The synthetic material is left in place until re-epithelization occurs; then it is gently removed, exposing the healed surface.

In the past several years, Acticoat (Westaim Biomedical, Exeter, N.H.), a silver-impregnated absorbent dressing, has been found to be useful in the treatment of partial-thickness burns. Its advantage is that the silver that is released provides antimicrobial activity against both gram-negative and -positive organisms.[13] It does not have to be changed more frequently than every 3 days. The Acticoat dressing is placed on the wound and is kept moist by applying sterile water, which activates the release of the silver ions into the wound in nanocrystalline form. An outer layer of gauze bandage such as Kerlix (Curad [Beiersdorf USA], Wilton, Conn.), or Kling (Johnson & Johnson Medical, Arlington, Tex.) is used to protect the wound and keep the Acticoat in place.

Use of Dressings

Burn wound dressings should be applied snugly to the injured area and should extend above and below the burn. They should be occlusive and have sufficient thickness or layers of gauze so that all the secretions are absorbed into the dressings. The purpose of the dressing is to protect the wound from bacterial contamination from the outside and to prevent the wound from rubbing against clothing or other objects. The frequency of dressing changes varies, depending on the amount of secretions. When antimicrobial creams are used, which require washing and reapplication, the dressings are changed once or twice daily. In the case of synthetic dressings such as Acticoat or Biobrane, however, dressing changes are required only once every several days as needed. The advantage to the patient of this type of dressing is the decrease in the frequency of dressing changes to once every 3 days or longer.

DEEP PARTIAL-THICKNESS (DERMAL) BURNS

Deep partial-thickness burns result from exposure to agents such as very hot water or hot oil. Upon presentation, the wound surface is less moist than in a superficial second-degree burn and is usually covered with an orange or light tan crust composed of dead collagen, which is very adherent to the underlying wound. The dead collagen must be completely débrided before healing can take place. Depending on their depth, these burns may require from 14 to 35 days to heal. Sometimes infection of the wound may destroy the remaining viable epithelium and cause conversion of the partial-thickness burn to a full-thickness injury. **Deep partial-thickness burns should be cared for by a burn specialist because enzymatic[14] or surgical débridement followed by grafting are often required.**[1]

FULL-THICKNESS (THIRD-DEGREE) BURNS

The dead skin covering the full-thickness burn is called an *eschar*. With the passage of time, the eschar of the full-thickness injury becomes permeable and loses the ability to control the rate of evaporation of water from the body.[15] An even more serious consequence of a full-thickness injury is that the skin ceases to function as a barrier against infection, and bacterial growth inevitably occurs in the deeper layers of the eschar. Depending on the extent of the full-thickness injury, the bacterial growth may become invasive and life-threatening septicemia may ensue.

Patients who sustain circumferential full-thickness burns of an extremity should be observed carefully. As edema forms in the subcutaneous tissues, a great deal of pressure is exerted against the eschar, which is stiff and unyielding. This may result in partial or even total occlusion of the blood flow to the extremity. The vessels to the distal extremities are especially vulnerable. The adequacy of the pulses to the extremities should be frequently monitored by a Doppler flowmeter.

If there is any question concerning the quality of the pulses with a circumferential extremity burn, an escharotomy should be performed. With IV sedation, escharotomies can be performed at the patient's bedside, using electrocautery to reduce the amount of bleeding. The incisions are made over the lateral and medial aspects of the extremities and of the digits in order to release the pressure exerted on the vessels by the edematous subcutaneous tissues (Fig. 16–4). **When the chest is involved by a circumferential full-thickness injury, escharotomies should be performed to improve the ease and completeness of ventilation.** These incisions are carried out in both anterior axillary lines. The incision of eschar should be carried out through the depth of the eschar into the subcutaneous tissues. When the compression is relieved, the subcutaneous tissue will pout out from the wound, and the arterial pulses will return to their normal levels. If they do not, and the burn is

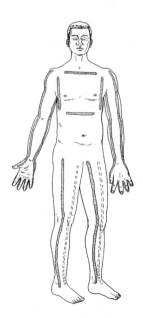

FIG. 16–4. Locations for incisions when performing escharotomies. (From Singer AS, Burstein JL, and Schiavone FM: Emergency Medicine Pearls, ed 2. Philadelphia, F.A. Davis, 2001, p 218, with permission.)

deep, or if there is a concomitant crush injury, the patient may have a compartment syndrome. In that case, the tissue pressures in the deeper compartment of the limbs should be directly measured. If the tissue pressures are elevated, they can be relieved in the operating room by releasing the fascia from its osseous attachments. **All patients with full-thickness burns should be managed by a burn specialist because the necrotic tissue needs to be surgically excised and grafted.** The proper timing of excision of the eschar depends largely on the overall condition of the patient.

ELECTRICAL BURNS

Electrical injury is caused by the passage of electrical current through the body. As the electric current encounters the resistance of the tissues of the body, it is converted to heat. The amount of heat produced is a function of both the amperage of the current and the resistance that that portion of the body offers to its passage. Thus, the smaller the size of the part of the body affected and the more bone there is in relation to the soft tissue, the more intense the heat becomes and the more damage occurs.[16] Thus, the fingers, feet, lower legs, and forearms suffer more extensive and devastating injury. The points of entrance and exit may usually be identified as necrotic areas, often several millimeters in diameter, that will heal by themselves. If they involve an area around the mouth or the fingers, however, an excision and extensive grafting or an amputation may be required. Delayed sloughing of the eschar at the corner of the mouth may result in significant bleeding from the labial artery in children who have bitten into an electrical cord.

The systemic effects caused by an electrical current depend on its voltage. A low-voltage current is defined as one below 1000 volts. Patients sustaining a low-voltage injury are in danger of developing an arrhythmia such as ventricular fibrillation. After such an injury, there may be nonspecific ST-T wave abnormalities on the electrocardiogram, and arrhythmias may also develop.

High-voltage injuries cause the most destructive tissue injuries. The muscles, fascia, and even bone are severely injured in the current's path. Such injuries are often life threatening and usually require amputations and very extensive operative excision of the injured tissues.

CHEMICAL BURNS

Chemical burns destroy the skin in such a manner that the depth of injury is difficult to assess. It is important to identify the causative agent because the destruction of the tissue can continue until the chemical is inactivated. Acid burns tend to be more limited in their depth than burns caused by alkali because alkali reacts with the fats in the skin, causing progressive injury.

Treatment of chemical burns begins with removing the causative agent as soon as possible. The chemical should be brushed off and washed by copious lavage with water for up 1 hour or until the pain subsides. Although the injury may initially appear to be superficial, it may become deeper after a few days; therefore, patients with chemical burns should be observed carefully for 4 to 7 days.

Hydrofluoric acid is frequently used in industrial settings, so patients with chemical burns from it are encountered from time to time.[17] If a substantial amount of hydrofluoric acid is absorbed into the body, it can cause arrhythmias as a result of the binding of the fluoride ion to calcium. The antidote is to inject calcium ions intra-arterially into the artery that perfuses the area affected. If this is not possible, then the injured tissue should be injected directly with calcium gluconate. For superficial injuries, calcium gluconate can be applied topically as a gel.

Another agent causing chemical burns is wet cement.[18] Inexperienced workers sometimes kneel in wet cement for long periods without protecting their knees, or the cement may enter their clothing and not be noticed for several hours. The wet cement converts to calcium hydroxide, and it is the alkaline hydroxyl ion that produces the injury. The resultant burn is treated in the standard manner.

Hot tar and asphalt can also cause severe burns. If a patient is exposed to hot tar directly from the container in which the tar is heated, it will cause a full-thickness injury. However, if an accident occurs from exposure to heated tar that has already been spread, the adherent tar must first be removed. It can be dissolved by applying a petrolatum-based ointment such as De-Solv-It. The wound is débrided by changing the dressings every several hours until the tar is dissolved and the wound becomes clean. The depth of the wound can then be properly assessed, and the wound can be treated in a manner similar to other burns.

REFERENCES

1. Brigham, PA, and McLoughlin, E: Burn incidence and medical care use in the United States: estimate, trends, and data sources. J Burn Care Rehabil 17:95–107, 1996.
2. Saffle, JR, Davis, B, and Williams, P: Recent outcomes in the treatment of burn injury in the United States: A report from the American Burn Association Patient Registry. J Burn Care Rehabil 16:219–232, 1995.
3. Moritz, AR, and Henriquez, FC: Studies of thermal Injury II. The relative importance of time and surface temperature in the causation of cutaneous burns. Am J Pathol 23:693–720, 1947.
4. Williams, WG, and Phillips, LG: Pathophysiology of the burn wound. In Herndon, DN (ed): Total Burn Care. WB Saunders, London, 1996, pp 63–69.
5. Arturson, G: Microvascular permeability to macro-molecules in thermal injury. Acta Physiol Scand Suppl 463:111–122, 1979.
6. Evans, EI, Purnell, OJ, Robinett, PW, et al: Fluid and electrolyte requirements in severe burns. Ann Surg 135:804–815, 1952.
7. Lund, CC, and Browder, NC: The estimate of area of burns. Surg Gynecol Obstet 79:352–358, 1944.
8. Fitzpatrick, JC, and Cioffi, Jr, WC: Diagnoses and treatment of inhalation treatment. In Herndon, DN (ed): Total Burn Care. WB Saunders, London, 1996, pp. 184–192.
9. Traber, DL, and Pollard, V: Physiology of inhalation injury. In Herndon, DN (ed): Total Burn Care. WB Saunders, London, 1996, pp 176–183.
10. Gimbel, NS, Kapetansky, DI, Weissman, F, et al: A study of epithelialization in blistered burns. Arch Surg 74:800–803, 1957.
11. Wheeler, ES, and Miller, TA: The blister and the second degree burn in guinea pigs: The effect of exposure. Plast Reconstr Surg 57:74–83, 1976.
12. Hinman, CD, Maibach, H, and Winter, GD: Effect of air exposure and occlusion on experimental human skin wounds. Nature 200:377–378, 1963.
13. Wright, JB, Hansen, DL, and Burell, RE: The comparative efficacy of two antimicrobial barrier

dressings: In-vitro examination of two controlled release of silver dressings. Wounds 10:179–188, 1998.

14. Soroff, HS, and Sasvary, DH: Collagenase ointment and polymyxin B sulfate/bacitracin spray versus silver sulfadiazine cream in partial-thickness burns: A pilot study. J Burn Care Rehab 18:253–260, 1994.

15. Caldwell, FT, Browser, GH, and Crabtree, JH: The effect of occlusive dressings on the energy metabolism of severely burned children. Ann Surg 193:579–579, 1981.

16. Sances, A, Mykelbust, J, and Larson, S: Experimental electrical injury studies. J Trauma 21:589, 1981.

17. Anderson, WJ, and Anderson, JR: Hydrofluoric acid burns of the hand: Mechanisms of injury and treatment. J. Hand Surgery 13:52–57, 1988.

18. Early, S, and Simpson, R: Caustic burns from contact with wet cement. JAMA 254:528–529, 1985.

JUDD E. HOLLANDER, MD

CHAPTER

17

Postoperative Care of Wounds

DRESSINGS

Postoperative wound care should optimize healing. It must be tailored to both the type of wound and the method of wound closure. Sutured or stapled lacerations should be covered with a protective, nonadherent dressing for 24 to 48 hours. **Maintaining a warm, moist environment increases the rate of reepithelization.** Hinman and Maibach[1] studied experimental split-thickness wounds in human volunteers who served as their own control subjects. They found that occluded wounds healed faster than those exposed to air; however, after 1 week, both groups were similar. On the other hand, leaving lacerations exposed to air does not affect the infection rate. Howells and Young[2] showed that the lack of postoperative dressings in 105 patients did not result in an increased infection rate. Therefore, maintenance of a moist wound environment with a dressing may improve healing, but it does not decrease the rate of infection.

Topical antibiotic agents should be used to maintain a moist environment in sutured or stapled lacerations but not lacerations repaired with tissue adhesive. Topical antibiotic ointments may help reduce infection rates and prevent scab formation. Dire and coworkers[3] compared topical antibiotics with petrolatum gel in 465 patients. They found that the infection rates with postoperative Neosporin or Bacitracin were one-third the infection rate of patients treated with petrolatum alone. Therefore, maintenance of a moist environment in sutured or stapled lacerations might be best accomplished by using topical antibiotic agents. However, patients whose lacerations are closed with tissue adhesives should not use topical ointments because they loosen the adhesive and may result in dehiscence.

Semipermeable films are manufactured from transparent polyurethane or similar synthetic films, which are coated on one surface with a water-resistant hypoallergenic adhesive. They are highly elastic, conform easily to body parts, and are generally resistant to shear and tear. They are permeable to moisture vapor and oxygen but are impermeable to water and bacteria. Common types of dressings are Opsite, Bioclusive, and Tegaderm. The disadvantages of these materials are that they cannot absorb large amounts of fluid and exudate and they do not adhere well in very moist states.

When possible, the site of injury should be elevated above the patient's heart to limit the accumulation of fluid in the wound interstitial spaces. Wounds with little edema heal more rapidly than those with marked edema. Pressure dressings can be used to minimize the accumulation of intercellular fluid in the dead space.

ANTIBIOTICS

Prophylactic oral antibiotics should not be used except for specific indications (see Chapter 18). Several studies[4] and a meta-analyses have all found no benefit to prophylactic antibiotics for routine laceration repair. Use of antibiotics should be individualized based on the degree of bacterial contamination, the presence of infection-potentiating factors (e.g., soil), the mechanism of injury, and the presence or absence of the host's predisposition to infection.[5] In general, decontamination is far more important than the use of antibiotics. Antibiotics should be used for most bites by humans, dogs, and cats; intraoral lacerations; open fractures; and wounds with exposed joints or tendons.[5] Additionally, patients with dirty soft tissue lacerations who are prone to the development of infective endocarditis, patients with prosthetic joints and other permanent "hardware," and patients with lymphedema should receive antimicrobial therapy. Patients at high risk for systemic complications such as endocarditis should be given intravenous antibiotic agents before wound care.

PREVENTION OF TETANUS

Tetanus status should be assessed before the patient is discharged. Two-thirds of the recent tetanus cases in the United States have occurred as the result of lacerations, puncture wounds, and crush injuries. For every wounded patient, information about the mechanism of injury, the characteristics of the wound and its age, previous active immunization status, history of a neurologic or severe hypersensitivity reaction after a previous immunization treatment, and plans for a follow-up visit should be recorded in a permanent medical record.

Proper immunization plays the most important role in tetanus prophylaxis. Recommendations on tetanus prophylaxis are based on the condition of the wound and the patient's immunization history. A summary guide to tetanus prophylaxis of the wounded patient is outlined in Table 17–1. Passive immunization with tetanus immune globulin (TIG) must be considered for each patient.

The only contraindication to tetanus and diphtheria toxoids is a history of

TABLE 17–1. RECOMMENDATIONS FOR TETANUS PROPHYLAXIS

History of Tetanus Immunization	Clean Minor Wounds		All Other Wounds*	
	Administer Td	Administer TIG	Administer Td	Administer TIG
< Three or uncertain doses	Yes	No	Yes	Yes
≥ Three doses				
Last dose within 5 years	No	No	No	No
Last dose within 5–10 years	No	No	Yes	No
Last dose > 10 years	Yes	No	Yes	No

*For example, contaminated wounds, puncture wounds, avulsions, burns, and crush injuries.
Td = tetanus-diphtheria toxoid; TIG = tetanus immune globulin.

neurologic or severe hypersensitivity reaction after a previous dose. Local side effects do not preclude repeated use. Local reactions, generally erythema and induration with or without tenderness, are common after the administration of vaccines that contain diphtheria, tetanus, and pertussis antigens. However, these reactions are usually self-limited and require no therapy. If a systemic reaction is suspected to represent allergic hypersensitivity, immunization should be postponed until appropriate skin testing is undertaken. If the use of a tetanus toxoid is contraindicated, passive immunization against tetanus should be considered in a tetanus-prone wound.

POSTOPERATIVE WOUND CLEANING

Sutured or stapled wounds should be gently cleansed after 24 hours. Goldberg and colleagues[6] demonstrated that the use of soap and water to cleanse lacerations was not associated with an increased infection rate. Gentle blotting should be used to dry the area. Wiping may result in dehiscence. Daily cleansing ensures that patients examine their lacerations for early signs of infection. Patients should be instructed to observe their wounds for redness, warmth, swelling, and drainage because these findings may indicate infection. Use of standardized wound care instructions improves patient compliance and understanding.[7]

Reapplying topical antibiotics continues to decrease scab formation, improving the likelihood of continued wound edge apposition. Patients with tissue adhesives may shower, but they should avoid bathing and swimming because prolonged moisture loosens the adhesive bond.

FOLLOW-UP

Patients should be told when and with whom to follow up for suture removal or wound examinations. Sutures or staples in most locations should be re-

TABLE 17–2. TIME FROM WOUND CLOSURE UNTIL REMOVAL OF SUTURES OR STAPLES

Location	Time, days
Face	3–5
Scalp	7
Chest	8–10
Back	10–14
Forearm	10–14
Fingers	8–10
Hand	8–10
Lower extremity	8–12
Foot	10–12

moved after approximately 7 days (Table 17–2). Facial sutures should be removed within 3 to 5 days to avoid formation of unsightly sinus tracts and hatch marks.[8] Sutures subject to high tensions (e.g., on the joints or hands) should be left in place for 10 to 14 days. When removing sutures, care should be taken to avoid applying tension in a direction that would tend to cause dehiscence. The suture should be cut on one side of the knot and then pulled out through the skin in the same direction (Fig. 17–1). Pulling out the suture in the opposite direction may result in wound dehiscence. Using a specialized curved stitch cutter and fine forceps helps ease removal of fine sutures. Any scab or crusting over the sutures may be débrided before suture removal by gently applying hydrogen peroxide with gauze.

To remove staples, the double-sided jaw of the staple remover is inserted beneath the exposed cross-limb of the staple. The upper jaw is then closed over the staple, elevating the ends of the staple and removing the staple from the skin (Fig. 17–2).

Tissue adhesives slough off on their own within 5 to 10 days of application. They do not require removal by a health care practitioner. When 2-octylcyanoacrylate is used, the patient should be careful to avoid picking at or scrubbing the area or exposing it to water for more than brief periods until healing has occurred. When tissue adhesives remain on the skin for prolonged periods, antibiotic ointment, Vaseline, or bathing can accelerate removal, but delayed sloughing is not necessarily a disadvantage. Acetone can be used when more rapid removal is required.

Healing lacerations and abrasions should not be exposed to the sun; exposure can result in permanent hyperpigmentation.[9] Abraded skin should be protected with a sun-blocking agent for at least 6 to 12 months after injury.

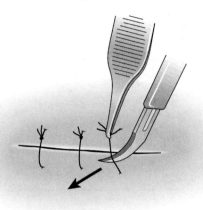

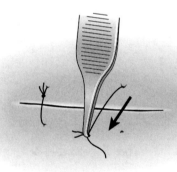

FIG. 17–1. Method of removing sutures. The suture is cut on one side of the knot and pulled out in the same direction.

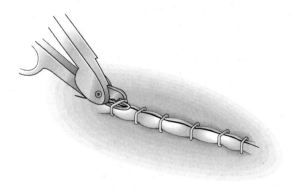

FIG. 17–2. Method of removing staples.

REFERENCES

1. Hinman, CD, and Maibach, H: Effect of air exposure and occlusion on experimental human skin wounds. Nature 200:377–378, 1963.
2. Howells, CHL, and Young, HB: A study of completely undressed surgical wounds. Brit J Surg 53:436–439, 1966.
3. Dire, DJ, Coppola, M, Dwyer, DA, et al: A prospective evaluation of topical antibiotics for preventing infections in uncomplicated soft-tissue wounds repaired in the ED. Acad Emerg Med 2:4–10, 1995.
4. Cummings, P, and Del Beccaro, MA: Antibiotics to prevent infection of simple wounds: A meta-analysis of randomized studies. Am J Emerg Med 13:396–400, 1995.
5. Singer, AJ, Hollander, JE, and Quinn, JV: Evaluation and management of traumatic lacerations. New Engl J Med 337:1142–1148, 1997.
6. Goldberg, HM, Rosenthal, SAE, and Nemetz, JC: Effect of washing closed head and neck wounds on wound healing and infection. Am J Surg 141:358–359, 1981.
7. Austin, PE, Matlack, R II, Dun, KA, et al: Discharge instructions: Do illustrations help our patients understand them? Ann Emerg Med 25:317–320, 1995.
8. Crikelair, GF: Skin suture marks. Am J Surg 96:631–632, 1958.
9. Ship, AG, and Weiss, PR: Pigmentation after dermabrasion: An avoidable complication. Plast Reconstr Surg 75:528, 1985.

GREGORY J. MORAN, MD
HANS R. HOUSE, MD

CHAPTER

18

Antibiotics in Wound Management

Although virtually all wounds are contaminated with bacteria to some extent, only a small fraction of them develop an infectious complication. Estimates of the incidence of infection of traumatic wounds vary tremendously, depending on the method of study and the population examined, but most studies[1] have found an incidence of 4 to 6 percent. **The best way to prevent wound infections is thorough wound cleansing and appropriate closure technique.** However, despite good wound care, some infections still occur. Antibiotics have an important role in the management of wound infections and may have a role in prophylaxis of certain high-risk wounds. **Appropriate choices for empiric treatment for most wound infections include a first-generation cephalosporin such as cephalexin or antistaphylococcal penicillin such as dicloxacillin. Patients with β-lactam allergies may receive a macrolide or clindamycin.**

This chapter discusses the optimal use of antibiotics in the management of patients with wounds and wound infections. The use of antibiotic agents for animal bites, plantar puncture wounds, and abscesses is discussed in Chapters 12, 14, and 15, respectively.

PRINCIPLES OF ANTIBIOTIC USE FOR WOUNDS AND WOUND INFECTIONS

EFFECTIVENESS

Activity against the likely pathogens is the most important consideration in choosing an antibiotic; other important factors include cost, convenience, and adverse effects. Because bacterial cultures require at least 1 to

194

2 days, treatment in the emergency department or office setting is almost never guided by culture results. A reasonable determination of the likely pathogens can be made, however, by considering the mechanism, circumstances of the wound, location on the body, and host factors.

The antimicrobial spectrum of a particular agent is determined by *in vitro* studies. This may not necessarily correlate with clinical effectiveness because simple *in vitro* sensitivities do not take into account the complex interactions of tissue fluids, fibrin coagulum, contaminated skin, the interaction of bacterial species, and the immune response. Most antibiotics in common use, including penicillins, cephalosporins, macrolides, aminoglycosides, and fluoroquinolones, achieve adequate levels in skin and soft tissues. Many antibiotics do not penetrate well into fluid collections and abscesses, so it is important that these infections be adequately drained. Aminoglycosides have especially poor penetration into abscesses, and their activity is inhibited by the low pH environment.

PRACTICAL ISSUES

Practical issues such as cost and dosing convenience must also be considered. Selecting a broad-spectrum antibiotic is usually not the best solution because they are typically more expensive (e.g., approximately $70 for a 7-day course of amoxicillin-clavulanate vs. $10 for a similar regimen of cephalexin) and may be more likely to select resistant organisms or cause adverse effects by disrupting normal flora. Antibiotics with more frequent dosing are clearly associated with lower compliance rates. Some drugs commonly used for wound infections, including cephalexin, cephradine, dicloxacillin, clindamycin, and erythromycin, have inconvenient qid (four times a day) dosing. Some physicians prescribe cephalexin 500 mg tid (three times a day) instead of 250 mg qid to simplify the regimen. Cefadroxil is a first-generation cephalosporin with bid (twice a day) dosing. Amoxicillin-clavulanate has traditionally been given tid, but the 875/125-mg dose can be given bid and appears to have fewer gastrointestinal (GI) side effects. Although some fluoroquinolones with once-a-day dosing are approved for treating infections of skin and soft tissue, they are generally not considered first-line agents because of their higher cost and because other agents are available that have greater activity against skin pathogens. In children, the palatability and dosing convenience of a drug can be very important in determining the success of a clinical regimen.[2] Dicloxacillin and erythromycin have been noted to have a bitter taste that may interfere with compliance.[3]

ADVERSE REACTIONS

Adverse reactions to antibiotics must also be considered. Fortunately, the β-lactam antibiotics preferred for most wound infections have a low incidence of adverse reactions, although some β-lactam antibiotics have more side effects than others. Diarrhea, for example, is reported by 9 percent of patients taking amoxicillin-clavulanate, but it is only rarely reported among users of cephalexin. Some newer formulations carry a milder side effect profile than their predecessors. Although erythromycin causes GI distress in approximately 20 to 25 percent of patients, azithromycin and clarithromycin have a much lower incidence of GI side effects as well as less frequent dosing.

EMPIRIC ANTIBIOTIC THERAPY FOR WOUND INFECTIONS

Gram-positive organisms such as *Streptococcus pyogenes* and *Staphylococcus aureus* are responsible for the large majority of wound infections. These are ubiquitous organisms that may be found in the normal flora of the skin, and they are introduced into any injury that causes a break in the integrity of the epidermis. Pathogens isolated from traumatic wounds have been found to be primarily the resident flora of the skin. Although recent bacteriologic surveys of traumatic wound infections are limited (most data in the literature focus on surgical wound infections), the few studies published confirm the predominance of these two pathogens[4,5]. *Staphylococcus aureus* has been found in about half of traumatic wounds; one-third yielded *Streptococcus pyogenes*, and 10 to 15 percent grew both organisms.[4] Gram-negative rods, enterococci, and anaerobes appeared in only about 10 percent of wound cultures. Although *Escherichia coli* has been found in as many as 25 percent of wound infections,[5] most studies have found a low incidence of gram-negative pathogens in uncomplicated infections.

First-generation cephalosporins (e.g., cephalexin, 250 to 500 mg every 6 hours), and antistaphylococcal penicillins (e.g., dicloxacillin, 500 mg every 6 hours) are appropriate therapy for most simple wound infections. In patients who are allergic to penicillin, the macrolide antibiotics erythromycin (250 to 500 mg every 6 hours), clarithromycin (500 mg every 12 hours), or azithromycin (500 mg once, followed by 250 mg/day), may be used. Clindamycin or the newer fluoroquinolones are alternative choices.

Most patients with simple wound infections can be safely treated as outpatients with oral agents. Occasionally, intravenous (IV) administration in an inpatient setting is indicated. Relative indications for admission include signs of systemic toxicity or underlying immunodeficiency states such as poorly controlled diabetes, renal failure, and chronic steroid use. Patients should also be considered for admission if they suffer a severe infection in a specific vital area (e.g., the face, orbit, hand, perineum, or lower extremity)—that is, any region that would result in disastrous morbidity if the infection continued to spread. IV therapy may also be warranted in suspected mixed flora or gram-negative infections. When treating patients with simple wound infections with parenteral medications, the drugs of choice are cefazolin (1 g every 8 hours), oxacillin (2 g every 4 hours), or nafcillin (2 g every 4 hours). All are reliably effective against both *Staphylococcus aureus* and *Streptococcus pyogenes*. Although some physicians are in the habit of adding penicillin to either oxacillin or nafcillin in order to provide better activity against streptococci, it is not necessary. As with oral therapy, alternatives for patients unable to tolerate penicillins or cephalosporins include the macrolides (erythromycin, clarithromycin, or azithromycin) and

TABLE 18–1. EMPIRIC ANTIBIOTICS FOR WOUND INFECTIONS

Clinical Situation	First-line Agent	Alternative Therapy	Comments
Uncomplicated cellulitis	First-generation cephalosporin or antistaphylococcal penicillin	Macrolide or clindamycin	
Patient with underlying immuno-deficiency	Amoxicillin-clavulanate or second-generation cephalosporin	Clindamycin plus a fluoroquinolone	Consider prophylaxis, especially in contaminated wounds
Patient with prosthetic heart valve or orthopedic implant	Consider adding vancomycin to standard regimen		Give prophylaxis when manipulating abscesses
Barnyard injuries; fecal contamination	Amoxicillin-clavulanate or second-generation cephalosporin	Fluoroquinolone plus clindamycin or metronidazole	Prophylaxis should be strongly considered
Saltwater exposure	Third-generation cephalosporin +/− doxycycline	Fluoroquinolone	*Vibrio* spp. may cause hemorrhagic, bullous lesions
Freshwater exposure	Antipseudomonal aminoglycoside or antipseudomonal penicillin	Fluoroquinolone	*Aeromonas* spp. or *Pseudomonas* spp. may be involved
Abscesses, infections due to IVDU	Amoxicillin-clavulanate or second-generation cephalosporin	Clindamycin	Antibiotics are usually not necessary; incision and drainage are essential
Necrotizing fasciitis	Ampicillin-sulbactam plus gentamicin plus clindamycin	Oxacillin plus ciprofloxacin plus clindamycin	
Bite wounds	Amoxicillin clavulanate or cefoxitin or cefotetan or penicillin and dicloxacillin	Azithromycin or ciprofloxacin plus clindamycin	Consider prophylaxis for high risk: Deep puncture, crush, hand injuries

(continued)

TABLE 18–1. EMPIRIC ANTIBIOTICS FOR WOUND INFECTIONS (Continued)			
Clinical Situation	**First-line Agent**	**Alternative Therapy**	**Comments**
Open fracture	First-generation cephalosporin or antistaphylococcal penicillin	Vancomycin	Add gentamicin for prophylaxis of severe open fractures
Plantar puncture wound osteomyelitis	Ceftazidime	Ciprofloxacin	

IVDU = intravenous drug use.

clindamycin. Vancomycin is not necessary for most wound infections, but it may be considered in persons with prosthetic heart valves, synthetic vascular implants, or orthopedic hardware underlying the infection. In these settings, coagulase-negative staphylococci may cause prosthesis infection.

Infections in patients with underlying diseases such as poorly controlled diabetes may call for more broad-spectrum antibiotics. Most acute wound infections in diabetic patients respond to the usual treatments such as first-generation cephalosporins or clindamycin. Serious or recurrent infections are more likely to be polymicrobial, with gram-negative and anaerobic organisms as well as *Staphylococcus aureus* and streptococcus. Agents such as amoxicillin-clavulanate or a combination of clindamycin plus a fluoroquinolone (with or without oxacillin) are appropriate.

Although most bacteria involved in wound infections originate from the patient's own body, exogenous pathogens may be introduced from the environment where the injury occurred and may require specific treatment in some circumstances. *Clostridium perfringens* or *Clostridium tetani* are associated with soil contamination, particularly in puncture wounds or those associated with crush injury. Wounds contaminated with animal or human feces (e.g., barnyard puncture wounds) are more likely to be infected with gram-negative enteric organisms and anaerobes.

Wounds with a history of marine or freshwater exposure are at risk for involvement of certain unique organisms. Marine exposures may be associated with infection from *Vibrio* spp., especially in patients with underlying liver disease.[6] Skin infections caused by *Vibrio* spp. tend to lead to hemorrhagic, bullous lesions and should be treated with ceftazidime with or without doxycycline or ciprofloxacin. *Mycobacterium marinum* may also be found with saltwater exposures. *Aeromonas hydrophila* or *Pseudomonas aeruginosa* may be seen in wounds exposed to fresh water. For serious infections resulting from freshwater exposure, consider adding an antipseudomonal aminoglycoside or fluoroquinolone to traditional gram-positive agents. Agents such as imipenem, meropenem, ticarcillin-clavulanate, or piperacillin-tazobactam may be used instead. Wounds that result from the handling of fish are at risk for the unusual pathogen *Erysipelothrix rhusiopathiae*. This organism responds to penicillin or ampicillin, and fluoroquinolones may be used in patients allergic to penicillin.[7] The recommended choices for empiric antibiotic treatment of wound infections are presented in Table 18–1.

NECROTIZING INFECTIONS

The most severe skin infections are deep, necrotizing soft tissue infections. These may initially be subtle in presentation, but they pose a significant threat to life and limb if not treated expediently. The tissue involvement is usually extensive and quickly spreading, but the classic signs of swelling, warmth, and erythema may not be present. The hallmark is crepitus on physical examination or tissue gas seen on radiographs, but these are late findings. Patients with necrotizing infections may present initially with severe pain and tenderness out of proportion to the physical findings. Systemic toxicity may be severe as the infection progresses.

Necrotizing infections are typically polymicrobial and should be aggressively treated; broad-spectrum antimicrobials such as a β-lactamase inhibitor combination plus gentamicin plus clindamycin is appropriate. The nomenclature of necrotizing infections is somewhat inconsistent and can be confusing. The terms *necrotizing fasciitis, monomicrobial necrotizing cellulitis,* and *Meleney's synergistic gangrene* are used to describe various types of necrotizing infections. As mentioned, most are polymicrobial and occur in patients with underlying chronic disease such as diabetes or renal failure. Organisms include *Staphylococcus aureus*, streptococci, and enteric gram-negative rods as well as a variety of anaerobic organisms. Necrotizing infections may occur after traumatic wounds, abdominal surgery, cutaneous ulcers, peri-rectal infections, and IV drug use. Fournier's gangrene is a variant of polymicrobial necrotizing fasciitis that occurs in the perineum.

Group A streptococcus (GAS), popularly known as "flesh-eating bacteria," can cause a rapidly progressing necrotizing infection in previously healthy individuals, sometimes after trivial trauma. This infection predominantly involves the subcutaneous tissue and fascia, with early sparing of the skin and only very late involvement of the muscle. Initially, the skin is painful but appears only mildly erythematous, and the area of involvement is not distinctly demarcated. As vessel thrombosis within the subdermal tissues occurs; the surface becomes mottled, edematous, or frankly necrotic; and blebs appear. After incision, thin, reddish-brown pus ("dishwater pus") may be released, and the skin may be found to be undermined.[8] GAS infections may also be associated with toxic shock syndrome.

Gas gangrene, or clostridial myonecrosis, results from a deep injury to skeletal muscle and leads to ischemia and tissue necrosis. Tissue gas can be found within muscle groups on radiographs. Toxins liberated by clostridial species infecting the wound can lead to profound systemic disease and mortality. A less severe form, known as *clostridial cellulitis*, has no muscle involvement and a more gradual onset.

Regardless of the specific syndrome involved, every necrotizing infection should be recognized as a life-threatening emergency. Immediate surgical consultation and broad-spectrum antibiotics must be initiated. Appropriate empiric antibiotics include a β-lactamase inhibitor combination plus an aminoglycoside or fluoroquinolone, imipenem, meropenem, or a combination such as oxacillin plus ciprofloxacin plus clindamycin. For GAS infections, animal data[9] suggest that a regimen that includes clindamycin may be superior to penicillin. This superiority is believed to be caused by a reduced efficacy of penicillin when large numbers of organisms are present as well as the ability of clindamycin to inhibit protein synthesis.

PROPHYLAXIS FOR WOUND INFECTIONS

TOPICAL ANTIBIOTICS

Although topical antibiotics such as mupirocin can be used successfully to treat patients with minor wound infections, the primary use of topical antibiotic agents is for the prevention of infection in fresh wounds. Topical ointments that contain bacitracin, neomycin, or polymyxin are routinely used by many physicians for fresh wounds. A survey[10] of emergency physicians in the United States found that 71 percent use a topical antibiotic on simple lacerations.

Despite the frequent use of topical antibiotic agents, there are surprisingly few studies that assess the efficacy of topical antibiotics on the suture line after closure. Animal studies[11] have shown that topical antimicrobial agents inside the wound before closure may reduce infection in contaminated wounds. One double-blind, randomized human trial[12] found a 5 percent infection rate with antibiotic ointment compared with an unexpectedly high 17.6 percent with petrolatum control. Other studies[13] have found no significant reduction in infection rates with topical antibiotics. Because the risk of infection is higher for crush injuries than for sharp lacerations, some experts recommend using topical antibiotics only for stellate wounds with abraded skin edges; however, this suggestion is not based on comparative trial data.

SYSTEMIC ANTIBIOTIC PROPHYLAXIS

Antibiotic prophylaxis is not necessary for uncomplicated wounds in immunocompetent individuals. Although it is tempting to prescribe prophylactic antibiotic agents to prevent wound infections, it is also important to note the limitations of this strategy. In many situations, the use of prophylactic antibiotic agents does not reduce the overall rate of infection, and it may also skew the bacteriology toward more unusual or resistant pathogens. To date, no randomized trials have demonstrated a benefit of antibiotic prophylaxis for simple wounds in immunocompetent patients.[14-18] A meta-analysis[19] of randomized trials has also confirmed the lack of benefit for simple wounds. Despite these data, it is still unclear whether there is a subset of high-risk wounds for which prophylactic antibiotics may be beneficial. Although it is known that certain types of wounds are more likely to develop infection, there is a paucity of good studies of prophylaxis for uninfected high-risk wounds. Many experts do recommend prophylaxis for some high-risk wounds. **Situations in which prophylaxis is sometimes recommended include an immunosuppressed host; an open fracture; a wound involving a joint, tendon, or cartilage; a grossly contaminated, high-risk bite wound (e.g., puncture, crush, extremity); an oral wound; or a significant delay before presentation** (Table 18–2).

TABLE 18–2. CONSIDERATIONS FOR PROPHYLACTIC SYSTEMIC ANTIBIOTICS
FOR WOUNDS

Immunocompromised host

- Poorly controlled diabetes mellitus
- Systemic corticosteroids or other immunosuppressants
- Renal failure
- Lymphedema
- AIDS

High-risk anatomical sites

- Oral lacerations
- Exposed tendon, bone, or joint
- High-risk wounds
- Large amount of crushed or devitalized tissue
- Heavily contaminated wounds, possible retained foreign body
- Some puncture wounds
- Many mammalian bites
- Significant delay before presentation

Immune Impairment

Prospective outcome studies[20,21] have found an increased infection rate in patients with immune impairment. Diabetes mellitus, malnutrition, renal failure, HIV infection, steroid use, chemotherapy treatment, extremes of age, and obesity have all been associated with more infectious complications. Patients with cardiac lesions at high risk for endocarditis should receive prophylactic antibiotics, as recommended by the American Heart Association, when undergoing procedures (e.g., the incision and drainage of a large abscess) likely to induce transient bacteremia. However, repair of a wound that is not grossly contaminated or infected does not require antibiotic prophylaxis.

Anatomical Site

The anatomical site of the wound may influence the risk of infection. Foot wounds appear to become infected more often than those involving other parts of the body, and injuries to the head and neck have the lowest rates of complication.[20] This disparity is often attributed to differences in regional blood flow, but greater contamination (both from environmental sources and endogenous flora) of lower extremity injuries is also important. A small, double-blind, placebo-controlled trial[22] of prophylactic penicillin for intraoral wounds found a trend toward possible benefit, most notably in patients with through-and-through wounds. Although hand wounds are often classified as high risk, studies[23,24] have failed to demonstrate a benefit of antibiotic prophylaxis for simple hand wounds. Most experts recommend prescribing prophylactic antibiotic agents for wounds in which tendons are lacerated or exposed. Although no randomized studies have been done in this group, it is reasonable to give prophylaxis for these high-risk injuries. Prospective studies have not been conducted to validate antibiotic prophylaxis for wounds involving the cartilage of the ear or nose, but this also seems appropriate. Open fractures or wounds into joint spaces typically require débridement and irrigation in the operating room in conjunction with the use of parenteral antibiotic agents. Minor open fractures of distal fingers appear to have a low risk of infection,[25,26] but prophylaxis should be considered for higher-risk patients.

Wound Mechanism and Contamination

The mechanism causing the wound may or may not influence the infection rate. Although some studies[27] have found that crush injuries are higher risk, presumably because of more devitalized tissue, which is impaired in its ability to resist bacterial growth, other prospective studies suggest that sharp and blunt mechanisms have similar rates of infection. The presence of collected blood within a wound acts as a growth medium and has been shown to increase risk of infection.[28] Wounds contaminated with more than 10^5 organisms per gram are at greater risk of infection, although there are no practical means to make this determination at the time of repair. Antibiotic prophylaxis should be considered for patients with wounds that are grossly contaminated and cannot be adequately cleaned. One of the most important local factors promoting infection is the presence of foreign bodies, including dirt, glass, metal, wood, bits of rubber or clothing, and even subcutaneous sutures.[29] Soft tissue gunshot wounds appear to be at low risk for infection and do not require antibiotic prophylaxis.

Delayed Presentation

Much has been written about the "golden period" of the time after injury in which a wound can be safely closed, and opinions differ as to when the increased risk of infection becomes significant. Although some studies (see chapter on wound assessment) have found that delayed closure does seem to influence the infection rate, several other studies[30] have shown that delayed closure (at least up to 18 hours after injury) does not seem to be a significant factor. Many experts recommend antibiotic prophylaxis for wounds with significantly delayed presentation, often in conjunction with delayed secondary closure.

Deciding on Prophylaxis

Although the available literature does not support the routine use of prophylactic antibiotic agents in all simple wounds and prophylaxis is poorly studied in high-risk subsets, it is reasonable to use prophylaxis in select settings. It is impossible to make generic recommendations that can account for the multiple factors present in any individual patient, so clinicians must use their own judgment. Prophylaxis should be *considered* in the situations shown in Table 18–2, especially if multiple factors are present.

Choice of Agents for Prophylaxis

The specific antibiotics used for prophylaxis are similar to those used for treatment of established infections. In most settings, a first-generation cephalosporin, antistaphylococcal penicillin (e.g., dicloxacillin), or macrolide is appropriate. Penicillin is an appropriate choice for intraoral wounds because of the activity against most common oral pathogens. Amoxicillin-clavulanate is the preferred prophylactic agent for high-risk bite wounds and for grossly contaminated, devitalized wounds in immunocompromised patients. Although many experts recommend a dose of parenteral antibiotics at the time of repair in order to quickly obtain high levels in the tissues, parenteral antibiotics have not been shown to be any more effective than oral antibiotics for wound repair.[14–18] For open fractures or joints, a parenteral antistaphylococcal agent should be given and an aminoglycoside should be added for severe open fractures. It is not necessary to give a prolonged course of antibiotics for wound prophylaxis; a 3- to 5-day course is adequate to reduce infection during the highest-risk period.

SUMMARY

Despite good wound care, some infections continue to occur. The choice of antibiotic for the prevention and treatment of wound infections is guided by the spectrum of likely pathogens, which can be surmised by considering the mechanism, circumstances of the wound, location on the body, and host factors. Other factors (e.g., cost, dosing convenience, and adverse effects) must also be considered. For most simple wound infections, activity against common gram-positive skin flora such as *Staphylococcus aureus* and *Streptococcus pyogenes* is important. Appropriate agents include first-generation cephalosporins, dicloxacillin, or macrolides. More broad-spectrum activity may be appropriate for more serious wound infections such as animal or human bites, wounds exposed to fresh water or other contaminants, or necrotizing infections.

Although the routine use of prophylactic antibiotics is not supported by the available literature, patients with certain high-risk wounds may benefit from antibiotics at their initial presentation. Situations for which prophylaxis should be considered include patients with significant immunocompromise; wounds involving bones, joints, tendons or cartilage; grossly contaminated wounds that cannot be adequately cleaned; high-risk bite wounds (e.g., puncture wounds, crushed or devitalized tissue, hand involvement); high-risk intraoral wounds; and wounds with a significant delay before presentation. The use of prophylactic antibiotics for puncture wounds to the foot is controversial.

REFERENCES

1. Hollander, JE, Singer, AJ, Valentine, S, et al: Wound registry: Development and validation. Ann Emerg Med 25:675–685, 1995.
2. Bauchner, H, and Klein, JO: Parental issues in selection of antimicrobial agents for infants and children. Clin Pediatr 36:201–205, 1997.

3. Steele, RW, Estrada, B, Begue, RE, et al: A double-blind taste comparison of pediatric antibiotic suspensions. Clin Pediatr 36:193–199, 1997.

4. Kontiainen, S, and Rinne, E: Bacteria isolated from skin and soft tissue lesions. Eur J Clin Microbiol 6:420–422, 1987.

5. Brook, I, and Frazier, EH: Aerobic and anaerobic microbiology of infection after trauma. Am J Emerg Med 16:585–591, 1998.

6. Morris, JG, and Black, RE: Cholera and other vibrioses in the United States. N Engl J Med 312:343–350, 1985.

7. Eron, LJ: Targeting lurking pathogens in acute traumatic and chronic wounds. J Emerg Med 17:189–95, 1999.

8. Lindsey, D: Soft tissue infections. Emerg Med Clin North Am 10:737–751, 1992.

9. Bisno, AL, and Stevens, DL: Streptococcal infections of skin and soft tissues. N Engl J Med 334:240–245, 1996.

10. Howell, JM, and Chisholm, CD: Outpatient wound preparation and care: A national survey. Ann Emerg Med 21:976–981, 1992.

11. Edlich, RF, Smith, QT, and Edgerton, MT: Resistance of the surgical wound to antimicrobial prophylaxis and its mechanisms of development. Am J Surg 126:583–591, 1973.

12. Dire, DJ, Coppola, M, Dwyer, DA, et al: Prospective evaluation of topical antibiotics for preventing infections in uncomplicated soft-tissue wounds repaired in the ED. Acad Emerg Med 2:4–10, 1995.

13. Caro, D, and Reynolds, KW: An investigation to evaluate a topical antibiotic in the prevention of wound sepsis in a casualty department. Br J Clin Pract 21:605–607, 1967.

14. Hutton, PA, Jones, BM, and Law, DJ: Depot penicillin as prophylaxis in accidental wounds. Br J Surg 65: 549–550, 1978.

15. Thirlby, RC, Blair, AJ, and Thal, ER: The value of prophylactic antibiotics for simple lacerations. Surg Gynecol Obstet 156:212–216, 1983.

16. Edlich, RF, Kenny, JG, Morgan, RF, et al.: Antimicrobial treatment of minor soft tissue lacerations: A critical review. Emerg Med Clin North Am 4: 561–580, 1986.

17. Day, TK: Controlled trial of prophylactic antibiotics in minor wounds requiring suture. Lancet 2:1174–1176, 1975.

18. Baker, MD, and Lanuti, M: The management and outcome of lacerations in urban children. Ann Emerg Med 19:1001–1005, 1990.

19. Cummings, P, and Del Beccaro, MA: Antibiotics to prevent infection of simple wounds: A meta-analysis of randomized studies. Am J Emerg Med 13:396–400, 1995.

20. Singer, AJ, Hollander, JE, and Quinn, JV: Evaluation and management of traumatic lacerations. N Engl J Med 337:1142–1148, 1997.

21. Cruse, PJE, and Foord, R: A five year prospective study of 23,649 surgical wounds. Arch Surg 107:206–209, 1973.

22. Steele, MT, Sainsbury, CR, Robinson, WA, et al: Prophylactic penicillin for intraoral wounds. Ann Emerg Med 18:847–852, 1989.

23. Haughey, RE, Lammers, RL, and Wagner, DK: Use of antibiotics in the initial management of soft tissue hand wounds. Ann Emerg Med 10:187–192, 1981.

24. Moran, GJ, and Talan, DA: Hand infections. Emerg Med Clin North Am 11:601–619, 1993.

25. Suprock, MD, Hood, JM, and Lubahn, JD: Role of antibiotics in open fractures of the finger. J Hand Surg 15:761–764, 1990.

26. Zook, EG, Guy, R, and Russell, RC: A study of nail bed injuries: Causes, treatment, and prognosis. J Hand Surg 9:247–252, 1984.

27. Cardany, CR, Rodeheaver, GT, Thacker, JG, et al: The crush injury: A high risk wound. J Am Coll Emerg Phys 5:965–970, 1976.

28. Krizek, TJ, and Davis, JH: The role of the red cell in subcutaneous infection. J Trauma 5:85–95, 1965.

29. Mehta, PH, Dunn, KA, Bradfield, JF, et al: Contaminated wounds: Infection rates with subcutaneous sutures. Ann Emerg Med 27:43–48, 1996.

30. Berk, WA, Welch, RD, and Bock, BF: Controversial issues in clinical management of the simple wound. Ann Emerg Med 21:72–80, 1992.

INDEX

Page numbers followed by an "f" indicate figures; page numbers followed by a "t" indicate tables; page numbers followed by a "b" indicate boxes.

Abscess(es), 53, 161–172
    antibiotics for, 162–163, 166–167
    definition of, 161
    differential diagnosis/
      management, 167–172
    drainage, 163–166, 164f–166f
    immunocompromised patients,
      167
    special considerations, 167–172
    treatment of, 162–167
Absorbable sutures, 60, 102t,
    104–105
Adhesive tape(s), 61, 64–71
    advantages and disadvantages,
      58t, 65t
    application of, 68–70, 69f–71f
    care of and removal, 71
    compared with sutures, 64–66
    contraindications, 66t
    history of, 65
    indications, 64, 66t
    mechanical properties, 67–68,
      67t
    See also Tissue adhesives
Allergy, 39
Anesthesia, 23–40
    for abscess drainage, 164,
      164f–165f
    allergies to, 39
    alternatives to traditional, 40
    clinical consideration in selection,
      38–40
    definition of, 45t
    dosing and toxicity, 38–39, 39t
    local, 23–26, 24t, 39
    regional, 23, 24t, 26–38, 27t
    See also Nerve block(s)
Animal bites, 133–138, 135t–137t,
    139t–140t, 142–145, 143t–144t
Ankle, 30–31, 34f

Antibiotics
    for abscesses, 162–163, 166–167
    adverse reactions, 195–196
    for bites, 136, 136t, 137t,
      139t–140t, 141–142
    effectiveness, 194–195
    empiric therapy, 196, 197t–198t,
      198
    for foreign bodies, 154
    for plantar puncture wounds,
      159–160
    postoperative, 189
    practical issues, 195
    systemic prophylaxis, 200, 201t
    topical, 200
    for wound management, 194–203
Anxiolysis, 43
Aseptic technique, 13–14

Bartholin's gland abscesses, 168
Benadryl. *See* Diphenhydramine
Benzyl alcohol, 40
Bites. *See* Animal bites; Human bites
Blades. *See* Scalpels
Boils, 168
Breast abscesses, 168
Burns, 173–186
    chemical, 185–186
    débridement, 54
    depth, 177–178
    dressings, 182–183
    electrical, 185
    extent, 176–177, 176f–177f
    fluid therapy, 178–180
    formation of edema, 175–176
    general principles of care,
      173–175
    immediate evaluation, 173–174
    inhalation injury, 180–181

Burns, (*Continued*)
  local care, 181–185
  patient age and, 174
  physiologic alterations after,
    175–176
  precautionary measures, 174
  tranfer to burn center, 174–175
Butylcyanoacrylate adhesives, 85t,
  92, 92f

Carbuncles, 167, 168
Cat bites, 135t, 137t, 138
Chemical burns, 185–186
Children
  burns in, 179f, 180
  human bites in, 140
  procedural sedation and analgesia
    for, 43t, 52–53
Chromic gut, 104
Clenched-fist injuries, 140
Computed tomography (CT), 151t,
  152
Conscious sedation, 44, 45t
Cosmetics, 5–7, 6f, 12
Crohn's disease, 171
CT. *See* Computed tomography
Cyanoacrylate adhesives, 83–96
Cytokines, 1, 2t

Débridement, 16–17, 17f, 54
Deep abscess extension, 171
Deep partial-thickness (dermal)
  burns, 178, 183
Deep peroneal nerve block, 33, 35
Deep sedation, 45t, 46
Dehiscence, 94–95
Delayed primary closure, 20
Diagnostic imaging studies, 150–152,
  151t
Diphenhydramine, 40
Dog bites, 133–138
  antibiotics for, 136, 136t, 137t
  bacteriology, 134, 135t, 136
  treatment, 136–138
Dog ear, 127–128, 129f
Drainage, of abscesses, 163–166

Drains, 20
Dressings, 182–183, 188–189

Edema, 99, 175–176
Electrical burns, 185
Escharotomies, 184, 184f

Face, 35–38, 35f–37f, 190
Felon, 169, 170f
Fentanyl, 49, 50t, 53
Field block, 165f
First-degree burns, 177–178, 181
Fluoroscopy, 151t, 151–152
Folliculitis, 167–168
Foot, 30–31, 33–35, 33f–34f
Foreign bodies
  clinical evaluation, 148–152
  diagnostic imaging studies,
    150–152, 151t
  documentation, 154–155
  exploration for, 149–150
  high-risk findings suggestive of,
    149t
  pathophysiology, 147–148
  potential complications, 148t
  removal, 54, 152–154, 153t
  treatment for, 152–154
  in wounds, 147–155
Full-thickness burns. See Third-
  degree burns
Furuncles, 167, 168
Furuncular myiasis, 171

Glycolide trimethylene carbonate, 105
Glycomer 631 sutures, 105
Granulation tissue formation, 4
Granulomata, 171
Growth factors, 3f

Hair removal, 14
Hand, 28f, 29–30, 29f–32f
Healing
  biology of, 1–7
  cytokines affecting, 2t
  stages of, 1–5

Hemostasis, 1, 15, 15f, 16f
Herpetic whitlow, 170
Hidradenitis, 168
Human bites, 138, 140–141

Immune impairment, 167, 201
Infection(s)
    abscess, 167–172
    anatomical site and, 201–202
    bite wound, 139t–140t
    empiric antibiotic therapy for, 196,
        197t–198t, 198
    foreign bodies and, 153t
    necrotizing, 171, 199–200
    prophylaxis for, 200–203
    risk of, 10, 11t
    sutures and, 98–99
    tissue adhesives and, 95
Inflammation, 1, 3, 153t
Infraorbital nerve block, 36, 37f
Inhalation injury, 180–181
Iontophoresis, 26
Irrigation, 17–19, 18f

Jet injection, 26

Ketamine, 49, 50t, 52, 53

Lactide sutures, 104
Lactomer glycolide sutures, 104
Lateral plantar nerve block, 31
Local anesthesia, 23–26, 24t
    allergies to, 39
    jet injection and iontophoresis, 26
    reducing pain of infiltration, 24–25
    topical, 25–26
Lymphogranuloma venereum,
    168–169

Magnetic resonance imaging (MRI),
    151t, 152
Marine infections, 198
Mattress sutures, 126–127, 127f, 128f,
    130f

Median nerve block, 29, 31, 32f
Medical history, 10–11, 46, 149t
Mentally challenged, 53
Mental nerve block, 36, 37f, 38
Metacarpal block, 28f
Midazolam, 48–49, 50t, 53

Necrotizing soft tissue infections,
    171, 199–200
Needle aspiration, 163
Needles, needleholders, 105–107,
    106f, 115f, 118f
    backhand approach, 117f
    choosing needle holder, 111
    holding needle holder, 111–112,
        112f, 116f
Neoplastic extension, 171
Neovascularization, 4
Nerve block(s), 24t, 26–38, 27t
    digital, 27–28, 28f, 29f
    of face, 35–38, 35f–37f
    of foot, 30–31, 33–35, 33f–34f
    of hand, 28f, 29–30, 29f–32f
Nitrous oxide, 51t, 52

Octylcyanoacrylate adhesives, 85t,
    92, 92f

Panacryl sutures, 104
Paronychia, 169, 170f
Patient assessment, 9–12
Physical examination, 11–12, 46, 149t
Pilonidal cyst abscesses, 168
Plain radiography, 150–151, 151t
Plantar puncture wounds. *See*
    Puncture wounds
Polydioxanone sutures, 105
Polyester sutures, 104
Polyglactin 910 sutures, 104
Polyglecaprone 25 sutures, 105
Polyglycolic acid sutures, 104
Polypropylene sutures, 100
Pott's puffy tumor, 170–171
Procedural sedation and analgesia
    (PSA), 42–54

Procedural sedation and analgesia
(PSA), (*Continued*)
definitions of sedation states, 45t
discharge after, 48
drugs, 44f, 48–49, 50t–51t, 52–54
indications, 43–44
monitoring, 47–48
personnel skills and training,
45–46
presedation evaluation and
preparation, 46–47, 47t
technique, 44–48, 47t
PSA. *See* Procedural sedation and
analgesia
Puncture wounds, 157–160

Rabies, 143–145, 144t
Radial nerve block, 30
Radiography, 150–151, 151t
Re-epithelialization, 3–4, 3f
Regional anesthesia, 23, 24t
See also Nerve block(s)

Saphenous nerve block, 33, 35
Scalpels, 110, 110f
Scars, 5–6, 6f
Scrubbing, 19–20
Second-degree burns, 178, 181–183
Skin antisepsis, 14
Skin hook, 108, 109f
Staphylococcus aureus, 196, 198
Staple(s), 60, 73–82
advantages and disadvantages,
58t, 79, 80t
aftercare, 81–82, 190
characteristics of staplers,
76t–77t
history of, 74
indications and contraindications,
80–81, 80t
removal, 81f, 82, 191t, 192
studies supporting usage, 73–75
technical aspects of usage, 75, 75f,
77, 78f, 79
Streptococcus pyogenes, 196

Superficial burns. *See* First-degree
burns
Superficial partial-thickness burns.
See Second-degree burns
Superficial peroneal nerve block, 33,
35
Supraorbital nerve block, 35–36,
35f–36f
Sural nerve block, 33, 34f
Surgical débridement. *See*
Débridement
Surgical needles. *See* Needles
Surgical staples. *See* Staple(s)
Surgical tapes. *See* Adhesive tapes
Suture(s), 59–60, 98–105
absorbable, 60, 102t, 104–105
basic techniques, 111–126
compared with adhesive tapes,
64–66
considerations in selection, 98–99
continuous dermal, 113t, 123–125,
124f–126f
continuous percutaneous, 113t,
120–121, 122f, 123, 123f
corner stitches and flaps, 130f, 131
deep, 121f–122f
edema and, 99
edges of uneven lengths and,
127–128, 129f
infection and, 98–99
interrupted dermal, 113t, 120, 121f,
124f
interrupted percutaneous, 112,
113t, 114–119, 115f–120f
materials, 100, 104–105
mattress, 126–127, 127f, 128f,
130f
nonabsorbable, 100, 101t, 104
nonlevel surfaces and, 129, 130f,
131
postoperative, 190
pros and cons of methods,
113t–114t
pros and cons of usage, 58t
removal, 99, 191f, 191t, 192
special situations, 126–132
See also specific types

Synthetic braided absorbable
  sutures, 104
Synthetic monofilament absorbable
  sutures, 105

Tapes. *See* Adhesive tape(s)
Tetanus, 143, 189–190, 190t
Third-degree burns, 178, 183–185
Tibial nerve block, 31, 34f
Tissue
  granulation, 4
  handling, 108–110, 109f
  undermining, 131–132, 131f
Tissue adhesives, 61–62, 83–96
  advantages and disadvantages,
    58t, 85–87, 86t
  application of, 88, 89f, 90, 90f–91f,
    92–94, 92f–94f
  clinical experience with
    cyanoacrylate, 84–85
  comparison of types, 85t
  indications and contraindications,
    87–88, 87t
  potential pitfalls, 94–95, 95t
  structure and properties of
    cyanoacrylate, 83–84
  wound aftercare and, 96, 96t
Topical anesthesia, 24t, 25–26

Ulnar nerve block, 29, 31f
Ultrasonography, 151t, 152
Undermining, 131–132, 131f

Vibrio infections, 171, 198

Whitlow, 170
Word catheter, 168, 169f
Wound(s)
  anesthesia, 23–40
  assessment, 9–12
  biology of healing, 1–7
  bites, 133–145, 143t
  burns, 173–186
  contraction and reorganization,
    4–5, 5f
  cosmetic outcome, 5–7, 6f, 12
  examination and exploration,
    11–12
  foreign bodies in, 147–155
  irrigation, 17–19, 18f
  postoperative care of, 188–192
  preparation, 13–20
  puncture, 157–160
  See also Wound closure
Wound closure, 56–62
  edges of uneven length and,
    127–128
  history of, 57
  methods of, 59t, 59–62
  nonlevel surfaces and, 129, 130f,
    131
  pros and cons of common
    techniques, 58t
  timing of, 56, 58–59
  See also specific means, e.g.,
    Suture(s)